**ABOUT THE AUTHOR**

After struggling with various eating disorders, **Alex Light** transformed her beauty and fashion blog into a digital safe space to help others. In doing so, she has opened up urgently needed conversations about eating disorders, weight stigma and diet culture, and she is passionate about using her platform to encourage change. Alex has a background in fashion and beauty journalism.

HQ
An imprint of HarperCollins*Publishers* Ltd
1 London Bridge Street
London SE1 9GF

www.harpercollins.co.uk

HarperCollins*Publishers*
1st Floor, Watermarque Building, Ringsend Road
Dublin 4, Ireland

This edition 2022

1
First published in Great Britain by
HQ, an imprint of HarperCollins*Publishers* Ltd 2022

ISBN: 978-0-00-850756-5

MIX
Paper from
responsible sources
FSC™ C007454

This book is produced from independently certified FSC™ paper to ensure
responsible forest management.

For more information visit: www.harpercollins.co.uk/green

Printed and bound in Great Britain by
Bell and Bain Ltd, Glasgow

This book contains descriptions of eating disorder thoughts and behaviours. If you are struggling with any of these issues you can contact the eating disorder charity BEAT in the UK (www.beateatingdisorders.org.uk). In the US, you can contact NEDA (www.national eatingdisorders.org) and in Australia, the Butterfly Foundation (butterfly.org.au). If you have concerns about your health, please consult a medical professional.

*Alex Light*

# YOU ARE not A BEFORE PICTURE

## How to Finally Make Peace With Your Body, for Good

# CONTENTS

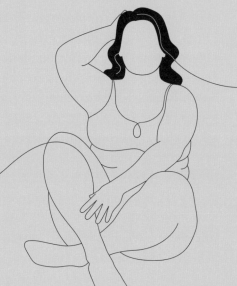
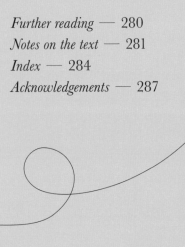

# I've spent far too long seeing myself as a 'before' picture

You know the one: the person with the slumped posture and sad demeanour in the infamous side-by-side shot waiting for the 'glow-up' (read: weight loss) that's guaranteed to make them happy, successful, admired and desired.

Growing up, I was bigger than my friends. Not fat, but chubby, and I was hyper-aware of it. I very strongly believed that there was something wrong with the way I looked, that it was holding me back, and this belief pushed me to start dieting around the age of 11. I dedicated the majority of my life from that point on to trying to achieve my 'glow-up', reducing my body – this powerful vessel that allows me to navigate the world – to a series of problem areas waiting to be fixed and shrunk.

I resent the amount of invaluable time, energy and money I spent doing countless diets over the years – Atkins, Dukan, South Beach, Mediterranean, Weight Watchers, Slimming World, Keto, Blood Type, Beyoncé's Lemonade diet (don't ask), Paleo . . . I could discuss them further but I'm reluctant to give them airtime because, quite frankly, they don't deserve the ink and paper. But you get the point: you name it, I've tried it. Pretty much every damn diet that existed before I broke free of dieting. As you're here, reading this, I imagine you might have a few to add to that list, given the amount of fads that have since emerged.

After some initial 'success' with a few (because diets do often offer very short-term success, which is why they can feel so irresistible) in my teens and early twenties, every single one of these diets ultimately – inevitably – left me miserable, despondent and utterly frustrated at myself for what I perceived to be my own failure. I wanted thinness more than *anything*, so why didn't I have the willpower to make it happen? It wasn't until years later that I would learn that it was never my fault, but we'll get on to that.

Growing up in a world dominated by diet culture, I was convinced that I needed to be thin to be liked, successful and worthy. All of the 'beautiful' people that existed in my world – brought to me courtesy of magazines, TV, film and pop music – were thin. I very strongly believed that I needed that too, not because I wanted to be on TV or be a popstar but because I thought that's how you gained approval and validation, and I was desperate for both.

Dieting became my personality, my entire sense of self, and my life revolved around it. I was a true chronic dieter, riding the fleeting highs and persistent lows and living off the hope I felt buoyed by when I discovered a new diet. My life was deeply impacted by this diet cycling: I avoided social situations that involved food for fear of slipping up and ruining the diet I was currently on, meaning that many of my relationships suffered, my work was average at best because I had finite headspace after dedicating so much precious time to 'staying on track' with what I ate, and I had limited energy because I was often depriving my body and brain of what it needed to function well.

Through sheer desperation, I began to make the diets more and more restrictive and ended up trying a juice diet. I was supposed to drink five juices a day as a replacement for food – which was incredibly painful; I distinctly remember desperately trying to go to sleep at 7pm to avoid the all-consuming hunger pains and sheer desperation to have food in my tummy – but I slowly found myself cutting this down to four glasses of liquid vegetables a day, then three, then two, then one . . . Until I decided that even that was too many calories and I settled on sucking boiled sweets to sustain me. I seemed to be unlocking a mental state even darker than my perpetual dieting and I was inching closer and closer to an eating disorder. I ended up needing treatment for anorexia nervosa and bulimia nervosa.

At the time, I was a fashion and beauty editor at a magazine. It was the job I'd always dreamt of and I'd worked hard to get there – I had interned for years in three different cities and sent out more CVs than you could shake a stick at – but I wasn't able to appreciate it: I was so desperately unhappy, because of my eating disorder, that I found very little pleasure in anything at that time. I also had an Instagram account with around 40,000 followers, all of whom were following me for my 'aspirational' fashion and beauty pictures. My life looked *so* glamorous but things really weren't what they seemed. I vividly remember a trip to Dubai in 2015 to interview Jessica Alba for a cover story. I was flown business class, put up in a five-star hotel, and wined and dined at some seriously swanky restaurants – my family, friends and followers couldn't believe it. I was the luckiest girl in the world! Nobody had any idea that I spent the entire trip going back and forth to bathrooms, desperately battling bulimia. On the flight home, having purged – made myself sick – for the fifth time and pulled a rib muscle in the process, I wondered if I was going to feel physically strong enough to lift my case off the baggage conveyor belt and get myself home from Heathrow.

Struck by my increasingly frail appearance not long after, in 2015, my poor, deeply concerned mum gently but firmly demanded I see a doctor. She referred me to a psychiatrist and that marked the beginning – but certainly not the end – of my damaging relationship with food and my body *finally* taking a turn for the better.

My recovery was long, hard and painful – as recovery from anything that has damaged us tends to be – and my initial diagnosis morphed into binge eating disorder before I eventually, years later, found true food freedom and body acceptance. But getting treatment and setting my sights on recovery was, hands down, the best thing I have ever done for myself.

I was lucky enough to be able to access professional help and my therapist opened my eyes to diet culture, this arbitrary world where I had lived my entire life, where nothing mattered as much as thinness and thinness was unquestionably the key that unlocked happiness. An all-pervasive ideology that was built and thrives for one reason only: it makes a lot of people in the diet industry a lot of money.

As I began to challenge diet culture – both inwardly, through challenging my deeply held belief that I needed to be thin, and outwardly, by acknowledging and debunking

the overwhelming amount of messages we are bombarded
with that tell us all bodies need to look a certain way to
be desirable, or just acceptable – I discovered a wonderful
alternative: the self-acceptance community.

In 2016, 'plus-size' model Iskra Lawrence shot to fame, making
headlines for shaking up the fashion industry and its lack of
diversity. I remember seeing her pictures and thinking how
beautiful she looked and how incredible it was to see a woman
who wasn't size 0 being chosen for campaigns and magazine
covers. I was tasked with interviewing her for a magazine
piece and met her at a restaurant to chat. She was stunning
– genuinely, one of the most beautiful women I had ever laid
eyes on – but it wasn't because of how much she weighed; it
was down to her confidence, self-assuredness and total lack
of apology for being herself. I could hardly keep my eyes off
her. The realisation that her beauty was about so much more
than how she – or her body – looked was strange for me and
it undoubtedly contributed to shattering a belief system I had
relied on since I could remember. I left the interview feeling
excited and inspired; I followed her on Instagram straight
away and, in turn, discovered a new whole online space full of
women who refused to bow down to society's beauty ideal and
were totally unapologetic about falling outside of it.

I have to admit that I found it hard to understand, initially
– I was confused as to how these women were so proudly
putting their (societally perceived) 'flaws', on display . . .
Did they *really* not mind them? I had spent most of my life
worrying about my cellulite, my thighs – did these women
*really* find their bodies acceptable? I don't know what images

of beauty you grew up surrounded by, but for me, it was undoubtedly and exclusively tall, thin, tanned white women with perfectly smooth, unblemished skin. While we are now, slowly, beginning to see more images of women whose bodies do not look like this, at the time, it was incredibly rare and it surprised me. I remember clearly thinking that I could never, ever show my body like these women were showing theirs.

The more of these images I consumed, the more I became desensitised and I began to see the beauty in them, questioning whether the 'flaws' were actually flaws . . . Because why IS cellulite viewed so negatively? Most women have it. Why are stomach rolls not OK? People *have* fat; they *have* skin folds. What is wrong with not having pin-thin legs? They fulfil their purpose pretty damn well, regardless of their shape and size.

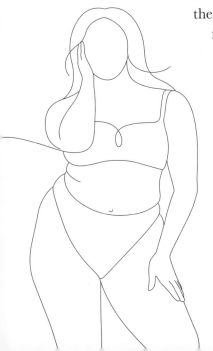

The more I questioned and challenged, the more I began to distance myself from body image pressures and what I now recognised as diet culture – and *not* an irrefutable law of what beauty has to look like. It was intentional but it also felt effortless – I found myself unable to align with anything that diet culture represented. I became invested in learning as much about it as possible and encouraging the women around me to break free from it, too.

This started off on a small scale – I have four sisters and, saddened by the huge role diet culture was playing in their lives, as well as my mum's, I started to pass on what I'd learnt. Seeing the positive effect that even considering dumping diet culture had on them propelled me to take it to Instagram.

When I was unwell and even well into my recovery, my account had only ever featured images that were heavily edited – I'm talking thinning, smoothing, blurring and the rest. Because, despite my newly acquired knowledge about diet culture, eating disorders, with their notoriously vice-like grip on the sufferer, don't tend to pack up and leave very easily with their body image concerns. But having those frank conversations about diet culture and body image with my family finally gave me the courage to take the plunge and make a change.

On 19 June 2016, I shared a post that detailed some of the weight and body struggles I had experienced throughout my life. It wasn't perfectly worded or explained – I don't think I had yet the capacity or knowledge – but it was a step in the right direction. The response was overwhelming: overnight, I received hundreds of messages from women who had similar stories. I was stunned to discover that so many were struggling with their body image, too . . . It wasn't just me. I had always thought it was just me.

Buoyed by the support, I felt compelled to continue. I slowly became more comfortable with being vulnerable and delved further and further into the story of my eating disorder and the body image struggles that had held me hostage my entire life. Any topic that I thought that might be helpful for someone suffering like I had, I researched and wrote about. My first viral post was about Bridget Jones – again, not worded perfectly; I still had a lot to learn. I explored how Renée Zellweger's character in the film was portrayed as fat and desperately in need of a makeover when neither was true. It was a narrative that had affected me – Bridget's weight was written across the screen and it was significantly lower than mine, yet she was depicted as 'overweight', something we're conditioned to fear over all else, and desperate to 'fix' herself (through calorie-counting and gruelling exercise – remember the exercise bike scene?).

Over the next few years, I must have had thousands of conversations with women all over the world about food, weight and body image through social media. I was asked to be on the digital cover of *Cosmopolitan* in early 2021, when they dedicated an edition to body confidence, and became a global ambassador for Dove, a beauty brand known for shaking up the industry with their 'Real Beauty' campaigns featuring women of different shapes and sizes. These were things I never would have dreamt of when I was suffering from an eating disorder and convinced that my only chance to make my body 'acceptable', and for me to be successful, was to make it smaller. The glaring irony being, of course, that lovely things started happening for me at exactly the point I broke free of this belief. I am at a much higher weight and the happiest and most successful I have ever been.

Having a thinner waist is not going to be your legacy, I promise.

I want you to be able to break out of diet culture, too. I would love for you to stop seeing your body as a 'before' picture, like I used to. It's hugely damaging to your mental health, often your physical health, too, and your wellbeing. If you're waiting until you've lost *insert random number of pounds/ kilos* to wear that dress or you think you'll go to the beach but only *after* getting rid of the cellulite then – and I'm sorry to be blunt – you're wasting invaluable time on an arbitrary goal that is unlikely to offer you true fulfilment. Despite what we're taught, real fulfilment only really comes from making a life that is meaningful – from building precious relationships and forming connections, pursuing passions, discovering your purpose, building a sense of self and living with compassion. Having a thinner waist is not going to be your legacy, I promise.

But where to start? Easier said than done, right?! Yep. I get it. I speak to women on Instagram every day who are desperate to improve their body image and ditch diet culture but . . . *how?* We have grown up in a world that teaches us to value thinness above all else, so to suddenly accept a body that sits outside of that category overnight is a tough ask. I'd go as far to say it's impossible. The answer certainly can't be boiled down to a single reply on Instagram, so I knew that this book was something I had to do. I believe wholeheartedly that it's only by learning the truth about diet culture and making peace with our bodies that we can move forward – and pass on that message to the next generation so that they don't struggle in the way that so many of us have.

I've always wanted quick fixes – welcome to my all-or-nothing brain that is a constant work in progress! – so getting to a place where I am happy in my own skin took a while – and it wasn't easy. I had to learn to swap my 'quick fix' plan for a 'jigsaw puzzle' approach. The individual pieces don't provide you with the full picture, an instant recipe for happiness and acceptance, but when they come together? They create something. Something magical, that makes sense.

So now it's time for you to tackle your very own jigsaw puzzle, and I've done my absolute best to fill this book with every piece you might need in order to get you feeling better in your own skin and quit dieting. We'll start with understanding and identifying diet culture, as well as challenging the effectiveness of dieting, before moving on to questioning our beliefs around thinness, fatness and health. We'll go on to cover body trends, comparing yourself to others, curating your space and how to put that all together in a way that works for you.

I speak from my own experience – some of which I share in these pages – and as someone whom I hope you will feel understands. However, I am not a nutritionist or a psychologist, so I have spoken to some experts in their field to further strengthen your understanding of the often complicated topics that come into the conversation around diet culture.

It would be wrong of me to not acknowledge the fact that I talk about body acceptance and anti-diet culture as a non-disabled, straight-sized, cis white woman. My body is not marginalised and I benefit from a great deal of privilege, which inevitably informs my understanding and experience of body image. For this reason, I have enlisted the voices of women whose bodies are marginalised to help educate us further on fatphobia, weight stigma and the oppression of marginalised bodies and, crucially, what we can all do to help.

I have tried to write the book that I so desperately needed back when I was obsessed with diets and giving up my social life to attend endless gym classes. When I believed that everything would be better if I was thinner and nothing would be enough if I wasn't. I'd like to think of this book as your body image bible, one that you can read, digest and put into action in your own time. And if one part doesn't seem to fit, that's OK – you can put it to one side, concentrate on other areas and come back to it when the picture is more complete and it might make more sense.

You bought this book for a reason. Use it. Because life is too short to hate the skin you're in.

# CHAPTER 1

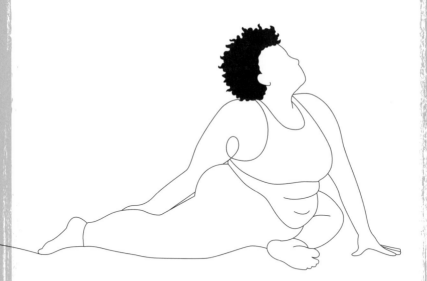

# Dismantling diet culture: a history of diets

# Diet starts Monday. Right?

And let me take a shot at guessing roughly how each week on a diet goes for you:

*Monday:* Determined. *So* determined.

*Tuesday:* I feel incredible . . . This diet is the one! It's going to work this time, I can feel it.

*Wednesday:* So full of energy! Nothing can stop me!

*Thursday:* I think I'm still good. Determined not to break it this time, but I *am* excited for a cheat day – I've got a list of everything I want to eat.

*Friday:* Bingeing on everything I've dreamt about eating during the week.

*Saturday:* Same as Friday.

*Sunday:* Same as Friday and Saturday but with an added layer of self-loathing, shame and disgust at myself for failing – again. Form a new plan for a new diet. *Next* week, it's going to be different.

**And so the cycle continues. Again, and again, and again.**

A poll of 2,000 adults commissioned in 2019 found that, on average, in the UK we try two fad diets a year, despite the fact that over half the respondents said they felt very confused over which diets were actually sustainable.[1] In other words, we're attempting to cut out all carbs, or sustain ourselves on cabbage soup or juice twice a year, every year, even though we don't know if it's going to work or not, so desperate are we to lose weight.

Of course, it never works, so we end up back on a Sunday, feeling full of that all-too-familiar shame, regret and sheer desperation. As I'm writing this, I feel as if I'm watching a slideshow of all the Sundays I have spent like this – the majority of Sundays of my life, undoubtedly. Isn't that sad? And even though I feel worlds away from that now, the flashbacks are visceral – I can *feel* that pain. It's all-consuming in its negativity and I'm suddenly reminded of how grateful I am to be free of dieting – and how important it is for you, too, to be free of dieting.

When I first started to interrogate diet culture, I became determined to understand it better – exactly what it is and where it's come from. I read everything I could about its origins and quickly started to see why it is so pervasive in our society today. I firmly believe that in order to dismantle diet culture and escape its powerful influence over us, we first need to understand it, and the root of that understanding is in its history. This knowledge will be an important piece of the armour that will shield you from it. So, bear with me as I take you on a journey – I promise it's fascinating.

## Firstly, what is diet culture?

Put simply, diet culture is a set of beliefs that puts thinness, shape and size above all else and equates it with health, success, happiness and moral virtue. Part of the way it does this is by glorifying a particular way of eating and demonising certain foods and food groups. The diet industry capitalises on these social narratives and the 'thin ideal' by selling products that claim to move consumers closer to it.

Let me expand – because there's a *lot* more I need to say about diet culture. The word 'diet' comes from the Greek *diaita*, which, in its original meaning, refers simply to a way of living, rather than a restrictive weight-loss regimen. And yet diet culture is rooted in the idea that being thin is the best and most morally superior thing a human can achieve, and therefore encourages individuals to stop at nothing to achieve thinness. It demands we devote precious time, energy and – crucially – money to shrinking our bodies, with a total lack of concern around the means used to do so or the ramifications.

It hasn't always been like this, though; for most of our existence, humans have been preoccupied with getting enough food to survive, not denying ourselves food in order to lose weight. For this reason, fat used to be a signal of wealth and health and it carried a higher social status – it equalled fertility and resistance to disease and famine, whereas thinness signified poverty, illness and potentially death. As a result, countless kings, pharaohs, gods and goddesses in the ancient world were depicted with fat bodies. Fatness is still considered desirable in certain parts of the world, of course – in many African cultures, being fat is a symbol of good life and wealth. In parts of Mauritania and Nigeria, girls and soon-to-be brides are even force-fed to make them plump and therefore 'attractive'. Perfect proof that the idea that thin is best/most attractive is simply conditioning and not an innate human preference.

So when did we, in the West at least, begin to see certain smaller body shapes as desirable and make associations between food and moral value? It's impossible to pinpoint exactly but we know that the Greek philosopher Hippocrates,

Diet culture is a set of beliefs that puts thinness, shape and size above all else.

considered to be the 'father of medicine', contributed to popularising the idea that fat = unhealthy and therefore 'bad' around 400BCE, writing, 'Sudden death is more common in those who are naturally fat than in the lean.'

What's thought to be the very first diet book came out in 1558: Luigi Cornaro was a 40-year-old fat Italian man who, tired of his size and inability to have sex, limited himself to 12 ounces of food a day and *14 ounces of wine*. His book, *The Art of Living Long*, advised others to do the same. Fourteen ounces of wine! I'm not sure what would be worse, my acid reflux or my vision . . .

In the early 1800s, poet, politician and self-confessed rake Lord Byron – who was also the premier male sex symbol in England at the time – was very vocal about his desire to stay thin, which saw him turn to extreme methods. He would starve, binge eat then try to 'sweat it off' under layers of clothing, eating nothing but either biscuits or potatoes drenched in vinegar. Eventually, he turned to drinking quantities of vinegar, combining this with water several times a day in an attempt to 'flush out' fat. The poet also openly condemned people – especially women – who ate what was, in his opinion, 'in excess'. Yuck. He was, of course, very unwell and in 2011, Professor Arthur Crisp, emeritus professor of psychiatric medicine at St George's Hospital medical school in London, said that he believed Byron suffered from 'severe anorexia nervosa'.

Diet culture turned another corner when British man William Banting decided to lose weight in 1862 due to health concerns and a growing cultural dislike for fatness. He found a doctor –

an ear, nose and throat specialist called Dr William Harvey – who agreed to assist him with an experimental diet that cut out all food containing starch and sugar and, in 1863, he wrote a booklet called *Letter on Corpulence, Addressed to the Public*, which detailed the particular plan for the diet he followed. It was incredibly popular and sold out several times – so many people followed it that the term 'I am banting' meant 'I am on a diet'.

The diet itself was low in carbs, and high in meat and fat. Similar to Atkins, but with six glasses of alcohol a day to help counteract the constipation accompanied by eating practically nothing but meat (seriously). In 2015, South African scientist Tim Noakes adapted the original diet and documented his version in a book titled *Real Meal Revolution* – the diet swept South Africa and soon there was at least one 'banting' option on countless menus across the country.

Banting's book recommended frequent weighing and, due to its popularity, scales to establish body weight soon became a collective preoccupation. By 1885, they were present in drugstores, pharmacies, train stations and even banks and offices, cementing a fixation on weight.

However, women in the Victorian era didn't aspire to be thin. The ideal woman's body was plump and hourglass-shaped: this was seen as highly feminine and a sign that their husbands could afford to feed them and care for them financially. The hourglass figure was achieved with the help of the corset, used to enhance a woman's curves by pulling in her waist. The corset was extremely popular but often

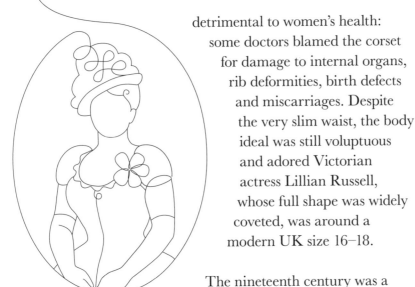

detrimental to women's health: some doctors blamed the corset for damage to internal organs, rib deformities, birth defects and miscarriages. Despite the very slim waist, the body ideal was still voluptuous and adored Victorian actress Lillian Russell, whose full shape was widely coveted, was around a modern UK size 16–18.

The nineteenth century was a time of fast progress in science and technology and the Victorians had a great appetite for novelty. So, unsurprisingly, fad diets came along with increasing pace and diet culture took hold. For example, in 1903, Horace Fletcher, an art dealer from San Francisco, was told he was too fat to qualify for insurance, so he invented his own weight loss plan – chewing each mouthful 32 times, or once for each tooth, and then spitting out the rest. 'Munching parties' became popular, where attendants stood around and counted their jaw movements up to one hundred. I'm half-amused, half-horrified by this visual . . .

The Industrial Revolution that began in the late eighteenth century brought about technological innovations that led to the mechanisation and mass production of clothing. Prior to this, the only way to get clothes was to visit a seamstress or make them yourself, both of which meant fitting the clothes to your body shape. In the twentieth century, we became used to cheaper, mass-produced clothes. Women in particular wanted to be able to buy affordable versions of the latest trends. But the 'problem' was – and always will be – that women's bodies come in all shapes and sizes. How could clothes be mass-produced to fit all of us? A move got underway to standardise sizing, driven by profit loss due to the need for alterations.

Measurements were taken to determine 'average' proportions of women and dress sizes were based on this. However, it was largely white women who were measured for this – troublingly, women of colour were excluded. So, starting from the 1950s, we got a version of the dress sizes we are familiar with today. Now, rather than clothes being made to fit your unique body, your body was expected to fit the clothes. This also gave us a simple metric for comparing our bodies with others and, you could argue, gave the world a useful tool for body shame.

*You can see how it's all starting to come together, can't you?*

In the West, there was a distinct racial aspect to our growing fascination with an 'ideal' body shape. Industrialisation also led to a significant surge of immigration as the factories needed a cheap source of labour. 'The emerging white middle class was looking for ways to assert and maintain a dominant position in relation to the new immigrants, and body size became a key point of comparison,' wrote registered dietitian and author

Christy Harrison in her book *Anti-Diet*. Increasingly, in the late nineteenth century, the middle class began to see thinness as an opportunity to cement their higher social status.

Charles Darwin published his book *The Origin of the Species* (full title: *On the Origin of Species by Means of Natural Selection, or the Preservation of Favoured Races in the Struggle for Life*) in 1858. Evolutionary theory, predominantly led by white men of Northern European descent, deemed white races more evolutionarily advanced and thus superior. Fatness was more identifiable in Blackness, therefore thinness was seen as more 'evolved' and, ultimately, more desired.[2] Essentially, fatphobia is rooted in racism. 'Discussions about racialised and gendered fat/slender bodies circulated largely in elite white space, and among white person, prior to the mid-twentieth century. They served as a mechanism for white men and women to denigrate the racially Othered body. They also worked to police and applaud the "correct" behaviours of other white people, especially white women,' wrote Sabrina Strings, PhD, in her book *Fearing the Black Body: The Racial Origins of Fat Phobia*. 'This is the crux of the issue. The image of fat Black women as "savage" and "barbarous" in art, philosophy and science, and as "diseased" in medicine has been used to both degrade Black women and discipline white women.'

Fatphobia and the cultural desire for thinness started to influence medicine, with doctors ultimately deeming fatness as 'unhealthy', despite a lack of scientific evidence to prove so. At the beginning of the twentieth century, health insurance companies began using the Quetelet index, which was later named 'the Body Mass Index' or BMI, to categorise people

Fatness was more identifiable in Blackness, therefore thinness was seen as more 'evolved' and, ultimately, more desired. Essentially, fatphobia is rooted in racism.

by weight. The categories were 'normal', 'overweight' and 'underweight' and the insurance companies began to associate excessive weight with decreased life expectancy based on some preliminary data that is widely considered dubious.

Let's go through a brief history of the Quetelet index while we're here. It was invented in the 1830s by a Belgian academic named Adolphe Quetelet as a method to test whether the laws of probability could be applied to human beings at the population level. It was derived from a simple maths formula and was never intended for clinical use on an individual formula. Furthermore, the method was based on statistics and data collected from European men, meaning that it didn't take into account different genders or races. We'll delve further into the reasons BMI is so imprecise (my preferred word here is actually 'bullshit' – let's see if I'm allowed to keep this in) in a later chapter.

The beauty ideal became significantly thinner than it ever had been, with women relentlessly being encouraged to lose weight. The advent of the 1920s 'flapper' signalled the end of the fuller figure of the Victorian era. Magazines started to print pictures of tall, thin women and the Western world subsequently began to covet a more slender, androgynous physique. Women turned to hiding their waists and wearing clothes that bound their breasts to create a flat-chested appearance.

Unsurprisingly, there were ever more 'experts' on hand to advise women on how they could force their bodies to achieve this newly desirable shape. Calories became formally recognised as a way to measure the energy value of foods in 1896; Dr Lulu Hunt Peters is thought to be one of the first people to count calories and to advise others to do the same. Her 1918 book, *Diet and Health with Key to the Calories*, which sold a staggering 2 million copies in 55 editions, advised women to stick to 1,200 calories per day, all eaten in 100-calorie portions.

This was, of course, around the same time that women won the right to vote in many countries, after a long and often brutal fight. Both Harrison and feminist writer Naomi Wolf believe this timing is far from coincidental: 'It's hard to smash the patriarchy on an empty stomach, or with a head full of food and body concerns, and that's exactly the point of diet culture,' wrote Harrison, while Wolf famously said: 'Dieting is the most potent political sedative in women's history; a quietly mad population is a tractable one.'

Shall we take a moment to think about that? Essentially, diet culture allows the patriarchy to thrive. I find it interesting that the era of thin, boyish flapper immediately followed women getting the vote and the 1980s obsession with aerobics and fad diets came after the strides made by the second wave feminists in the 1960s and 70s. Keeping women busy with body concerns is one way of making sure they stay quiet and obedient – of keeping them shrinking, literally and metaphorically. Does this make you angry? Because it makes me angry – angry that I wasted so much time preoccupied with how my body looks that I did indeed stay quiet and obedient – but also determined. Determined to help wake as many others as possible up from this oppression and reinvest their energy in things that are truly going to have a positive effect on their lives.

Keeping women busy with body concerns is one way of making sure they stay quiet and obedient – of keeping them shrinking, literally and metaphorically.

*Apologies – I got carried away.
Back to history!*

Despite the lack of sufficient data surrounding the theory that higher weights correlated to poor health, the diet industry was fast growing and promised to line the pockets of many, so it quickly became an unchallenged fact. Weight-loss products had begun to take off from the late Victorian era, with laxatives, soaps that 'wash fat away', compression garments and tapeworms (yes, tapeworms – one would swallow a tapeworm or tapeworm pills, the worm would then live in your stomach and consume some of your food. I simply cannot . . . ) being advertised in magazines and newspapers. Diet pills became very popular – generally containing amphetamine (speed) or an amphetamine derivative at best, iodine, arsenic and other poisons at worst. In the mid 1930s, hundreds of thousands of pills that contained dinitrophenol, a highly toxic industrial chemical, were sold, but many who tried it went blind or even died, and by 1938 it was designated as 'not fit for human consumption'. Women began to enjoy more social freedoms in the 1920s and 30s, including smoking in public, which had been taboo. Cigarette companies were thrilled and marketed cigarettes as health aids that benefitted digestion and helped smokers to stay slim.

The 1920s also saw the arrival of the Golden Age of Hollywood, arguably one of the strongest influences on beauty standards. Americans were able to visit their local movie theatre to watch short silent movies starring impossibly glamorous, thin women like Greta Garbo and Clara Bow. There was some pushback against dieting in this period, with doctors speaking out against dangerous diet products and the new beauty standard of thinness, but the diet industry continued to grow regardless, with brushes, chewing gum, bath oil and drinks all promising to provide weight loss. From dangerous to ridiculous, I swear diet culture runs the gamut, never leaving a stone – or possible money-making opportunity – unturned.

The 1930s produced many diets still peddled today, like the Body Ph and the Grapefruit Diet, also known as the Hollywood diet. The latter consisted of eating half a grapefruit with each meal, followed by not much else; it is founded on the claim that grapefruit has a fat-burning enzyme. Another popular diet to come out of the thirties was the Alkaline diet: founded by Dr. William Hay, it involved dividing all foods into alkaline, acid or neutral and claimed you shouldn't combine acid and alkaline. There is no scientific evidence to back up his claims, yet the alkaline diet still exists today – Gwyneth Paltrow is long-reported to be a fan.

There was a slight dip in diet culture frenzy in the early 1940s due to the Second World War and food rationing, with people being encouraged to finish all the food on their plate. But it soon picked back up, with magazines offering exercise routines alongside suggested diets. The Lemonade Diet (or 'Master Cleanse'), where you drink nothing but one teaspoon each of lemon juice and maple syrup with cayenne pepper in a glass of water six to twelve times a day, became popular and the first ever weight loss support group was formed. Esther Manz created TOPS – Take Off Pounds Sensibly – in 1948 for people who wanted to get together, discuss their mutual food struggles and track their weight.

Marilyn Monroe emerged as the 1950s epitome of beauty: fuller-figured and curvy, she became the ultimate pin-up and, yet again, the ideal shifted. This sparked a new demand for the perfect hourglass shape – tiny waists and big busts. Diet advertisements started to air on television, as did group exercise programmes, and this decade also saw the first ever bariatric surgery (weight loss surgery). It had been devised to be used in rare, urgent cases, but physician Howard Payne saw a way to make money: he coined the term 'morbid obesity' in an attempt to paint the surgery as lifesaving (because, you know, 'morbid' doesn't sound great, does it?).

By 1959, TOPS had 30,000 members. But in 1961, housewife Jean Nidetch founded the most famous dieting group to date, Weight Watchers, after gathering a group of friends in her house to talk about weight loss. She was frustrated with her yo-yo dieting past and was eager to lean on support from others. Within five years of its launch, Weight Watchers, with its points system for calculating calories, had a staggering 5 million members worldwide.

Following Marilyn's celebrated hourglass physique of the 1950s, the desired body began to slim down, but there was a noticeable shift in the 1960s when British fashion model Lesley Lawson, known as Twiggy, shot to fame. Twiggy, who was only still a developing teenager at the time, made waves in the fashion industry for her waif-like, androgynous figure and she became the face – and body – of the 1960s. Women all over the world now coveted this look but it was incredibly hard to attain for the vast majority. Hence a more urgent desire to lose weight, which resulted in even more new and far-fetched diet products: a liquid shake called Metrecal, which was to replace meals, came onto the market (the taste of which was often likened to 'baby sick' – yum). Elvis Presley, known for his weight struggles, tried the Sleeping Beauty Diet, which involve taking sleeping pills and being unable to eat for a few days while you were unconscious (not sure I have words for that one). Garments like corsets and binding materials were replaced by diet and exercise and the incidence of women being admitted to hospital for anorexia nervosa rose significantly.[3]

Slimming World was founded in 1969 in a church hall in Derbyshire by Margaret Miles-Bramwell, characterised by a system that divided up foods into categories like 'free foods', 'healthy extras' and 'syns'. Diet pills were still very popular and by 1970, 8 per cent of all prescriptions were for amphetamines.

The 1970s saw the rise of fat-liberation groups, who worked hard to debunk the myths around weight, health and the efficacy of dieting. The National Association to Advance Fat Acceptance, or NAAFA, was founded in 1969 and the organisation worked hard to address weight bias and discrimination against fat people as a civil rights issue, while the Fat Underground was founded in the early 1970s by

Thin remained the ideal and diet culture continued to dominate, with more and more diets, diet products and diet groups available …

… along with wildly inaccurate nutritional information to support the various diets.

a group of women in Los Angeles as a radical offshoot of NAAFA. The group asserted that American culture fears fat because it fears powerful women and tirelessly sifted through medical journals to find statistics and studies that proved the widespread fatphobia it identified in the medical establishment. The organisation disbanded in 1983 but it was responsible for paving the way for the ensuing fat liberation activism.

Despite their efforts, thin remained the ideal and diet culture continued to dominate, with more and more diets, diet products and diet groups available, along with wildly inaccurate nutritional information to support the various diets.

In 1972, cardiologist Robert Atkins published *Dr Atkins' Diet Revolution*, a book that detailed a compelling case against eating carbs. It was revolutionary in the sense that you did not have to count calories or limit how much you were eating, as long as you were eating the 'right' foods: poultry, meat, butter, cheese, fats and oils. Nuts and salad greens were to be introduced in later stages of the diet. The diet caused a stir and, at the height of its popularity, one in eleven Americans were on Atkins.

But the tide turned in the 1980s, with dieters reverting to a low-fat approach for weight loss, and diet food products reached their peak, with supermarket shelves lined with 'low-calorie' or 'low-fat' options (the fat had been replaced by starches and sugar and were substantially less filling). A notable dieting moment from the 1980s came in the form of Oprah Winfrey dragging a wagon holding 67 pounds of fat across the stage on her TV show to represent the weight she lost on a liquid diet. (She gained the weight back once she started to eat food again.)

Jane Fonda helped shift the focus from skinny to strong, as her aerobics became an international craze. Supermodels like Cindy Crawford, Christine Brinkley and Elle MacPherson embodied the 'perfect' body of this era with their tall, toned and athletic physiques. Long, lean legs and broad shoulders became highly coveted and shoulder pads were the defining fashion must-have of the decade.

Supermodels stormed the early 1990s, with Linda Evangelista, Naomi Campbell and Christy Turlington representing the body *du jour* – tall and thin, yet still athletic and curvaceous. Despite not meeting the normal height criteria for models, thin, willowy, 17-year-old model Kate Moss skyrocketed to fame in the mid-1990s during the (frankly horrifyingly named) 'heroin chic' era – a style characterised by pale skin, dark under-eye circles, emaciated features, androgyny and unkempt hair. Meanwhile, low carb was back – the Atkins diet from the 1970s resurfaced and reached new levels of popularity with the release of *Dr Atkins New Diet Revolution* in 1992. Atkins low-carb products could be found in most supermarkets, alongside a host of other diet options, such as calorie-portioned popular snacks like crisps and biscuits.

*Notice the diet culture pattern of demonising different food groups?!*

Fat's bad, then carbs are the devil, then sugar is the real villain – and then we cycle back through them all over again . . .

In 1994, the American Psychiatric Association recognised anorexia and bulimia and added 'eating disorders, non-specified' to their list of mental disorders, but binge eating wasn't to be recognised until 2013. Pamela Anderson first appeared in *Baywatch* in her iconic red bikini in 1991 and the girl-next-door look combined with large round breasts became the ideal for many. By the early 2000s, it was all about boobs and breast implants had become increasingly popular, with glamour model Katie Price undergoing a series of operations that took her up to a size 32GG. (Pamela Anderson has since said she regrets her own breast augmentation.)

The 2000s saw diets like South Beach, Paleo, Medifast and Dukan – basically, a less extreme version of Atkins – become popular. I tried all of them, of course and (spoiler alert!) none worked. Well, I lost a lot of weight on Atkins but I developed a grey tinge to my skin and people around me started to ask whether I was OK. I wasn't really – I was eating blocks of cheese and double cream and mounds of meat and I simply couldn't sustain it for longer than a few weeks. As soon as I started eating carbs again – and I did so with a vengeance, I was desperate – I gained back the weight and more.

Meanwhile, diet pills were still being sold but, luckily, their ingredients were not as toxic or dangerous as they had been in previous decades and now contained natural stimulants like green tea and acai berries. In 2009, the FDA approved Alli as effective for weight loss – a drug containing active ingredient orlistat, which interferes with how you digest fats: as well as not actually working, this caused digestion issues for many (uncontrollable bowel movements were a very common complaint). Fitness gadgets also became popular, with wearable electronic devices calculating calories, carbs and protein intake, as well as sleep patterns and calories burned.

The media took a sinister turn in the late 1990s into the 2000s and it was open season on women in the public eye. Celebrities like Britney Spears, Paris Hilton, Nicole Richie and the Spice Girls were regularly attacked in the press: they were upskirted (upskirting refers to the act of taking a photograph beneath a person's dress/skirt without their permission – it only became illegal in the UK, following a tireless campaign from British activist Gina Martin, in early 2019) by paparazzi as they got into cars and the pictures printed. These young women were photographed relentlessly to try to capture 'bad' angles and their bodies were scrutinised daily.

Victoria Beckham was weighed by Chris Evans on *TFI Friday* just 12 weeks after giving birth. 'Is your weight back to normal? Can I check?' he asked, pulling out a pair of scales. 'Oh no, you did this to Geri, didn't you?' a visibly flustered Victoria protested, referring to her bandmate who publicly suffered from bulimia. 'Oh come on, come on,' he encouraged, before weighing her and having the camera zoom in to reveal that she was eight stone. It's still, to this day, one of the most horrifying displays of body image I've ever seen on TV. 'Eight stone's not bad at all,' he said.

The scrutiny of these women's bodies undoubtedly had a hugely negative effect on the women themselves, and also us, the people constantly consuming this overt body shaming.

Nicole Richie, on the other hand, was on the receiving end of intense media shaming for being Paris Hilton's 'fat' friend on *The Simple Life* (she wasn't fat – at all). She went on to drop a significant amount of weight and was labelled anorexic: 'Nicole Richie's Weight Plummets in HORRIFYING Skin-and-Bones Photos' read a particularly cruel headline. Nicole has always denied the rumours of an eating disorder, it's important to note.

The scrutiny of these women's bodies undoubtedly had a hugely negative effect on the women themselves, and also us, the people constantly consuming this overt body shaming. With our body insecurities at an all-time high, juice diets became popular in the 2010s, with followers replacing all food with fresh juices, as well as more high-tech options to attempt to lose weight, like DNA kits, bought online, which were sent off and returned with a personalised diet. The Blood Type Diet, popular among Hollywood stars like Demi Moore and Courtney Cox-Arquette, and the Metabolic Type diet, were other fads that became mainstream during this decade.

Despite the diet industry showing no signs of abating – think laxative teas marketed as 'Flat Tummy Tea', 'SkinnyJab' weight loss injections and gastric band balloons that can be swallowed to expand in the stomach – many started to grow disillusioned with dieting in the mid 2010s thanks to the rise of the body positivity movement and the anti-diet culture movement. And some began to loudly say what, on some level, we had always known. These diets didn't work. Not in any meaningful way. With a multibillion-dollar industry at stake, diet culture rebranded to keep up, pivoting to using terminology like 'wellbeing' and 'lifestyle', rather than 'weight' and 'diet'. In 2018, Weight Watchers changed their famous brand name to WW, with new tagline, 'Wellness That Works'.

Weight-loss app Noom launched in 2016, marketing itself as a 'lifestyle change' that implements long-lasting behavioural change, with the tagline, 'Stop dieting. Get life-long results.' It is cleverly branded as weight loss 'designed by psychologists' that uses a psychology-based approach to change eating habits 'for the better'. It has tricked many – I have spoken to countless women on Instagram who believed this could *finally* be the solution to their weight loss desires, before realising it is just another diet dressed up in fancy clothes. It is, essentially, a calorie tracker, using a traffic light system to 'rank' foods according to the calories they contain, yet it is valued at $3.7 billion – this staggers me. But it shouldn't surprise me: the diet industry knows it has a captive consumer and is deft at adapting so that it continues to trick so many people into losing precious time, energy and money with a promise it can never keep.

We still live in a culture obsessed with thinness and it fuels the diet industry. I often talk about how to eliminate diet culture from our lives but I think the truth is that it is not fully possible, living as we do in a world where it is so pervasive. Diet culture is everywhere, at every turn: from colleagues or friends discussing their latest weight-loss attempts to compliments about weight loss and constant advertisement for products/diet programmes/exercise equipment that tell us we are not good enough if we are not trying to be thinner.

Diet culture is pretty much white noise to me at this point and I don't tend to take much notice, but I recently made a point of spending one day being as observant of it as possible and writing everything down – here was my list:

- I woke up, checked Instagram and saw a before and after picture of Adele's weight loss, with the caption: 'So inspirational!!!'

- Went to a gym class, saw a sign that read: 'Summer body transformation in eight weeks: sign up now!'

- Got lunch from a shop in town and spotted the 'low calorie' options for 'healthier choices'.

- WhatsApped with a friend, who said she was 'being good' because she had a wedding coming up and wanted to get into a certain size dress – so no carbs for her for the foreseeable.

- Watched a video on YouTube, got served a Noom ad.

- Ate a snack that read: 'only 98 calories' on the packet, front and centre.

- Scrolled TikTok before bed, saw one ad for intermittent fasting and one ad for gym leggings to get rid of cellulite.

You get my point! It's *everywhere*. And it's no wonder it's so pervasive – as we've discovered, diet culture has been with us for a *long* time. It's rooted in history and ingrained in the fabric of our society, so it's not our fault that we are also entrenched in it. If you feel bad about your body or if you have been a chronic dieter like me, that's not on you – but it's time for us to rebel.

We might not be able to get rid of diet culture completely *but* we can build up a personal armour against it so that when we encounter it, we're able to let it bounce off rather than internalise it, allowing it to inform our beliefs about ourselves and our own bodies. We can't let it take any more of our power away from us. The first step to building that armour is understanding it and how it came about, so, congrats – first step taken! You have the first piece of the puzzle. Now you know exactly what diet culture is, and where it came from, it's time to learn the truth about diets . . .

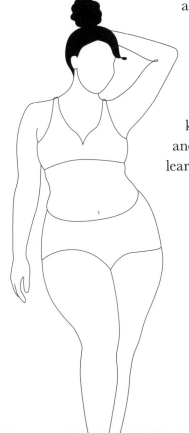

# CHAPTER 2

'The definition of insanity
is doing the same thing over
and over and expecting
different results.'

**ATTRIBUTED TO ALBERT EINSTEIN**

# The ugly truth: diets don't work

# CHRONIC DIETERS

A chronic dieter is an individual who consistently restricts their food consumption to manipulate their weight. If you yourself are not a chronic dieter, you'll almost definitely know one. These are some of the red flags that might indicate chronic dieting:

- Being 'good' every Monday.

- Knowing exactly what you weigh.

- Tracking everything you eat.

- Always tempted by the next new diet.

- Separating how you eat into 'good' and 'bad' categories.

- Eating 'clean' in the week and bingeing over the weekends.

- Wanting to talk to others about their diets.

- Interest in knowing what others weigh.

- Having 'cheat' days.

# How many times have you been on a diet in an attempt to lose weight?

I'd love for you to take a minute to think about what that number might be. Got it? Now, think about how many of those attempts resulted in sustained weight loss . . .

I'm going to hazard a guess that that answer is 'none', given the purported efficacy of dieting: the statistic often quoted is that 95 per cent of people who lose weight on a diet will gain it back.

Though, it's worth saying that this statistic has been frequently challenged by people in the diet culture space, and not without reason. It originally came from a 1959 study by Dr Albert Stunkard and Mavis McLaren-Hume that looked at just 100 people in an 'obesity' clinic who were living in larger bodies and had chronic battles with their weight and eating. In the words of Stunkard, they 'were just given a diet and sent on their way' without any supervision. Ninety-five of the hundred participants ended up at the same starting weight or higher, hence the 95 per cent conclusion.

So it's quite reasonable to ask why this number is still being quoted as a fact, so many years after this tiny study was carried out. But there have been other, more recent studies into the effectiveness of dieting. Traci Mann, a psychology professor at the University of Minnesota, and a team of researchers did a painstaking review of every subsequent study that followed people on weight-loss programmes for two to five years. The results? Although dieters in the studies had lost weight in the first nine to twelve months, over the next two to five years, the majority had gained back all of the weight – and some even more. Their conclusion was that between one and two-thirds of dieters will regain more weight than they originally lost.[4]

'You can assume that the first six to twelve months are the weight-coming-off part, and then after that is the weight-coming-on part,' said Mann. In her book, *Secrets from the Eating Lab*, she writes: 'Anybody who says, "On this diet, it's just going to come off and not come back" is lying. There's no such diet. That's just not the way it works.'

Still unsure? Let's take this study of twins by Pietiläinen et al. carried out in 2011.[5] It observed 4,129 individual twins born in Finland between 1975 and 1979. Their weights and heights were recorded at ages 16, 17, 18 and 25 years old, along with the number of intentional weight loss episodes of more than 5kg at 25 years. The results suggested that the more intentional weight loss episodes, the higher the individual's susceptibility to weight gain. Both identical and non-identical twins who dieted where their sibling didn't ended up heavier than their twin on average. In summary, the researchers concluded that dieting makes you prone to gaining weight in the future. Read that again.

*Dieting is actually counterproductive for weight loss.*

Let's also consider some evidence of a more anecdotal nature: if diets worked, every person would only need to do one in their lifetime. It would be a success and they wouldn't need to diet again, right? The diet industry certainly wouldn't be worth $192.2 billion and you probably wouldn't be reading this book right now.

Imagine if any other product had such a sky-high failure rate: people wouldn't dream of wasting their money, time and energy investing in it. And what if not only did it fail to deliver on its promise but it actually did the exact opposite? Imagine a washing up liquid, for example, that left your plates even dirtier than when you started or an iron that added more creases to your shirt – it's a ridiculous idea, isn't it?! And yet that's where we are with the products we are being sold by the dieting industry.

So let's consider the reasons why diets don't work. When I embarked upon diet after diet, there was never a lack of motivation and enthusiasm: in fact, I wanted weight loss more than *anything*. I was so determined, so why couldn't I achieve it? Why wasn't I able to push through and get the results I so desired? Why did I feel so weak and lacking in willpower?

*I wasn't. I know now that it was never my fault. And it's never been yours.*

'The industry has sold us a lie,' says registered dietitian Lauren Cadillac (@feelgooddietitian on Instagram). 'It tells us that if we just try hard enough, if we have enough "willpower"

Dieting makes you prone to gaining weight in the future.

Read that again.

and "motivation", then we can all be thin. But there are several issues with this: firstly, our weight is largely determined by our genetics. Much like your eye colour, height and shoe size, we have a set point weight range that is genetically predetermined – some folk are genetically predetermined to have smaller bodies, while others will have larger bodies. Our set point weight is the weight you maintain when you are eating intuitively, honouring your hunger and fullness cues and engaging in joyful movement.'

So shrinking our bodies is difficult in the first place, thanks to our genes. But there are other factors at play, and Cadillac suggests observing the Minnesota Starvation Experiment to explore these. This landmark study was carried out by physiologist Ancel Keys in 1944 and was designed to determine the physiological and psychological effects of severe and prolonged dietary restriction. At the time, the world was still gripped by the Second World War and hunger and starvation were widespread, but there was little research into its effects on the mind and body.

The experiment chose 36 young men who were all in good physical and mental health, and began with a three-month period during which the men consumed 3,200 calories per day, their maintenance calories, for three months. For the six months immediately after, the men had their calorie intake nearly halved to 1,570 per day in order to lose 25 per cent of their normal body weight, along with physical activities like walking 22 miles per week and laboratory duties.

Their mental health suffered in the starvation period, with reported mood and personality changes including depression, irritability and apathy, and the men developed an all-consuming obsession with food – they struggled with intense cravings, collected recipes ('stayed up until 5am last night studying cookbooks,' recorded one participant, according to *Men and Hunger: A Psychological Manual for Relief Workers*, that described the initial findings) and conversation revolved around food. But the starvation period affected their physical health, too: their metabolism dropped by 40 per cent. 'As you can see, the effects of restriction mimic the effects of dieting,' says Cadillac, 'with increased thoughts of food, cravings, bingeing and mood changes.'[67]

A refeeding period followed, where the men were allowed to eat whatever they wanted. I'm pretty sure you can guess what happened next: their preoccupation with food continued and they experienced extreme hunger, some bingeing on thousands of calories at a time and others finding it difficult to stop eating. While around three months later, the subjects' moods stabilised, there remained lasting effects on their eating, with continued bingeing reported among several participants. 'Not only do diets flat out not work, but they cause physical and psychological harm,' says Cadillac. 'The Minnesota Starvation Experiment is proof of this.'

Cadillac explains the results of this study from a biological standpoint: 'If we take a very brief look at history, throughout our existence as a species, humans have experienced famine and food scarcity. Our bodies have learnt how to adapt and protect ourselves from these famines. If food is scarce, the human with more energy reserves (fat) is far more likely to survive than the human with less energy reserves, right? Learning to make and store fat in times of famine is a matter of human survival. What our body doesn't realise is that, for the majority of folks (food insecurity certainly still exists and the level of privilege for folks that are able to practise intuitive eating without this barrier should be highlighted), there is a grocery store around the corner. It doesn't realise that, when we restrict our calorie intake, a *true* famine is not occurring but rather a *self-imposed* one.

'As we saw in the Minnesota Starvation Experiment, dieting leads to increased thoughts about food. Have you ever gone on a diet and found yourself daydreaming over what you're going to have at your next "cheat meal"? Or maybe you find yourself watching food porn or just thinking about food constantly: this is no coincidence. This is your body's way of trying to get your attention and have you seek out food.'

Wow. This has unlocked many memories: towards the beginning of when I was restricting, I would be utterly obsessed with food. I remember walking past restaurants in Soho and just stopping to take in the delicious smells of foods and see what people had ordered. As my restriction continued, though, I became fearful of this preoccupation with food – I worried it was going to lead to me losing control and bingeing, so I purposefully avoided walking past restaurants or watching adverts on TV in case they featured food and I unfollowed anyone who might post food pictures on Instagram.

But why? Why does our body obsess over food when it doesn't have enough of it? In order to further explore the physical aspect of this, let's refer back to the idea of a set point weight. 'Our body works hard to keep things like body temperature, fluid balance, blood pH and blood sugar within a specific range,' says Cadillac, 'and it also works hard to regulate the amount of body fat we have – a region of our brain, known as the hypothalamus, plays a large role in maintaining our bodies' set point weight range. If your body starts dipping below your set point, the hypothalamus will signal the body to slow down metabolism while simultaneously increasing appetite.'

Appetite is increased by various hormones and chemical messengers and many are increased during periods of fasting or restriction – it's our brains telling our bodies that resources are running low and we need to eat. An example of this is neuropeptides, which stimulates our desire to eat, particularly carbohydrates. So, by the time you *do* eat, you're likely to find yourself eating beyond comfortable fullness – but NOT because of self-control, because of biology. And there we have it. Diet culture glorifies willpower but our biological instincts trump willpower every time – and that's a *good* thing. Acting on willpower actually means overriding and rejecting your body's genuine needs and wants, but we're not supposed to be disconnecting emotionally from our body.

So here's how it goes when you break your diet: you feel like you've failed, you're upset at yourself, you berate yourself for a lack of willpower. But here's what *actually* happens: your body says, 'Thank you! I hated what you were doing to me and I was desperately trying to tell you. Promise I know best.'

*You paid attention and honoured your body by breaking the rules.*

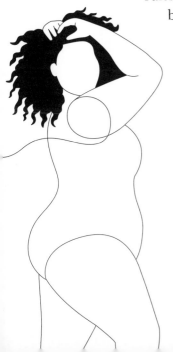

Imagine how it would feel to be totally free from rules and completely connected to your body? I distinctly remember the period when I stopped dieting. I woke up and felt sheer joy and relief at the idea that I was going to be able to eat breakfast – it sounds so simple and minor, but after my lifelong rule that I didn't eat before 1pm in order to 'save' calories for later on in the day, this felt incredibly joyful. Eating breakfast (along with an increased calorie consumption) felt liberating – and the benefits were immediate: I had energy, I was far less grumpy and I felt much, much happier.

Imagine how it would feel to be totally free from food rules and completely connected to your body.

My body was saying: 'Yes! At last! It only took 30 years . . . '

Thirty years! Eek. So much time spent at war with my own biological instincts – with the serious consequence of developing an eating disorder, which is, unfortunately, *not* a rare consequence of dieting. According to the National Eating Disorder Association (NEDA), those who engage in moderate dieting are five times more likely to develop an eating disorder, while those who engage in extreme dieting are 18 times more likely to develop an eating disorder. Bearing in mind that anorexia nervosa has the highest mortality rate of any psychiatric disorder, this shows how diet culture can be fatal.

There are, of course, a number of factors that contribute to an eating disorder – most people who simply try a diet won't go on to develop an eating disorder. While scientists can't say for sure what exactly causes an eating disorder or predict who might develop one, most experts agree that they are complicated illnesses that arise from not just one cause but from a complex combination of biological, psychological and environmental factors. I am, therefore, by no means saying that they are all caused by dieting, but if someone is already predisposed to developing one, dieting is only going to cultivate it and give it the means to thrive.

I believe that's what happened in my case – I have many of the distinct personality traits that scientists have identified as common in individuals with eating disorders, like perfectionism, all-or-nothing thinking, a drive for order and symmetry, doubt and worry (and yes, I know what you're thinking – I am indeed the life and soul of a party). So the susceptibility was there but diet culture sealed the deal. I grew up in a diet culture-heavy environment, as is the case for most of us, where thinness was admired, adored and celebrated. I picked this up from a young age and made it my mission to achieve it. The result being multiple eating disorders and an incredibly unhealthy relationship with food and body image.

I hope that this hasn't been your experience too, and if it has then I am so sorry. The truth is that to be on a diet is not only damaging to your own physical and psychological wellbeing but also to that of those around you. I didn't just learn that thinness was the ultimate aspiration from magazines and the TV when I was growing up – the message also came from those around me, as of course they too had been negatively impacted by diet culture. Diet culture has a ripple effect and its impact stretches far and wide. For this reason, it's imperative we eliminate it not only from *our* lives, but from the lives of the younger generations – too many of us grew up with overt diet culture that continues to plague us. If I have children, I vow to avoid referring to any body – including my own – in a negative light, to teach them about diet culture so they understand it and to provide them with tools to identify it and dismantle it themselves, so they can approach food and eating with neutrality.

But even for me, someone who is now significantly informed about diet culture, that will require effort, because diet culture has disrupted our relationship with our bodies and food to a point where harmful things go totally unquestioned and unchallenged in society every single day. Let me dive into an example briefly: it is extremely common to describe foods as 'good' or 'bad', for example. You know, 'good' food like vegetables (unless they're potatoes, of course) and 'bad' food such as chocolate, pasta and white bread.

We've all heard it: 'No thanks, I'm being good today,' while turning down a piece of cake. 'I'm being so bad,' while eating a doughnut.

But assigning a moral value to food and eating cultivates a culture of shame around both, which fuels disordered eating and eating disorders. And it's also classist – 'bad' foods are generally cheaper than 'good' foods, and using such terminology further marginalises people whose choices around what they can eat are limited by inequalities, such as income and education.

And here's the thing: food is not good or bad. Food is food. Treating yourself to a doughnut does not mean you have questionable morals and going for carrots and hummus over a bag of crisps as a snack does not make you any more decent as a human being. Yes, some foods are more nutrient-dense than others and some foods should be consumed less than others for a variety of reasons. But the black-and-white thinking about food, as either virtue or vice, is a diet culture trick that ends up having the opposite of the intended effect: avoiding a specific food or food group will only lead you to, ultimately, crave it even more.

A phrase I heard when I was beginning my recovery from my binge eating disorder always stuck with me: 'When you deprive, it thrives.' This simple, five-word phrase unlocked

Diet culture has disrupted our relationship with our bodies and food to a point where harmful things go totally unquestioned and unchallenged in society every single day.

something I could never understand: I wanted so badly to stay away from things like cakes and biscuits and crisps – why did I always end up gorging on them? Because they were my 'off-limits' foods and being so aware of the fact that they were off-limits made me crave them until I could no longer resist. You get my point: all signs point to it – diets don't work. Not only has this been scientifically proven – and shown by our own experience – but we also categorically know that they cause psychological and physiological harm to us, breed a culture of shame and harm those around us, and future generations.

*Looking at these simple facts alone, it seems unthinkable that diet culture remains so pervasive, doesn't it?*

And if this was the whole story perhaps we would easily be able to shrug off the whole sorry mess, leaving juice cleanses and grapefruit diets behind us. But there is, of course, a whole other factor in play that helps keep it alive . . .

# CHAPTER 3

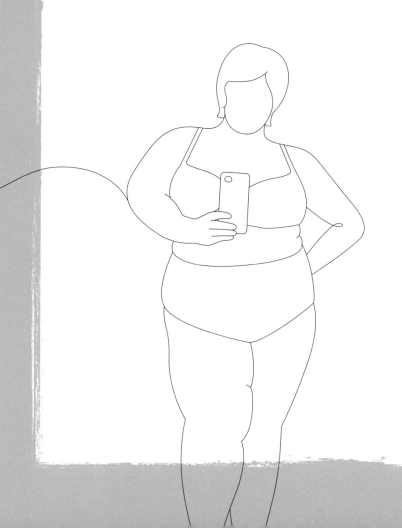

The media
have a lot
to answer for

If I ask you to conjure up the image of a 'beautiful' woman, what do you picture?

When I was growing up, the ideal beauty standard that I saw everywhere – on TV, in adverts, in magazines – was someone young, tall, thin, white or light-skinned, with curves 'in all the right places' (boobs and bum) but minimal fat on her stomach or limbs, with long, lean legs, flawless long hair and perfect make-up. And while things are getting better in terms of representation, I think most of us would agree that this is still far too prevalent in mainstream media.

*But . . . why? How has this standard come to be widely seen as 'typically beautiful'?*

It's largely down to the mainstream media, which perpetuates a scarily narrow standard of beauty by showing *only* this type of beauty and holding it up as the ideal. Think about a typical magazine: the front cover features either a model or a glamorous, thin celebrity – both heavily airbrushed and edited – and inside, you'll find a plethora of beautiful women accompanied by articles centred around the importance of physical appearance, including weight discussion, which is usually also featured on the front page. One particularly troubling edition was from *Shape* magazine in 2013: Britney Spears was on the front page, surrounded by the following snippets of text: 'Drop 10lbs FAST!', 'Tighten Your Tummy', 'Britney – 31, Firm and Fabulous' and 'Get it now! A Body Built for Sex!'. From 2012 to 2016, only 9.4 per cent of *Vanity Fair* covers included a non-white subject. *Harper's Bazaar* managed to go for 17 months without including someone of colour on the cover, from September 2013 to February 2015.[8] And even when people who are non-white are featured on the cover of glossy magazines, they overwhelmingly tend to be thin, young and non-disabled.

Not to mention the scrutiny of women's bodies laid out in painstaking detail: as recently as 2021, magazines have run features entitled 'This Year's Best & Worst Beach Bodies – The Good, The Bad & The Ugly!'. The subtitle? 'From fab to flab, celebs let it all hang out!' The 'good' bodies are accompanied by adjectives such as 'toned', 'banging', 'red-hot' and 'beautiful', while the 'bad' bodies are described with words like: 'whale', 'sight for sore eyes', 'flabby', 'saggy' and 'lumpy' (the *National Enquirer*, 2 August 2021).

This form of abuse has been rife in print for decades, with most of it going totally unquestioned . . . by me, too. I distinctly remember, when I was in the thick of my body image hell, picking up magazines and flicking straight to those sections, desperate to discover that my body didn't look as bad as the 'bad' bodies; the idea that the magazine would ridicule and denigrate my body in a similar way if they had pictures felt unbearable. If I did see a 'bad' body that looked similar to mine, I punished myself with extra starvation and restriction. And I wasn't the only one to be affected by print media: a 2007 study that followed 2,500 girls in secondary school found that those who were heavy readers of magazines were twice as likely to engage in disordered weight control behaviours.[9]

Then you look at television and film, both of which feature almost exclusively 'beautiful' people with lean bodies –

Only around
5 per cent of
women possess
the body type
typically shown
in the media.

How does that
leave the other
95 per cent of
people feeling?

successful, fat actresses are very rare, but we'll get onto that in a minute. Advertising? The same: typically beautiful person after typically beautiful person. Anything that strays even slightly from that almost induces shock in the consumer because we are so conditioned to see one type of beauty.

For generations, the media has been a significant contributing factor to a negative body image, though it's not the only one. Body image is a term used to describe how we perceive, think and feel about our bodies, and it's formed by a combination of sociocultural factors, including our experiences with our bodies in the world (e.g. our interactions with other people), our intrinsic beliefs (formed according to the culture we live in) AND the media that we are exposed to. But the mass media represents by far the most powerful and persuasive influence[10] and this is at the very least in part explained by the fact that the media helps to set standards which inform these experiences and intrinsic beliefs . . .

Essentially, the media has a lot to answer for. Reinforcing key messages that we need to conform to an 'ideal' in order to be successful, healthy and desirable has harmed us as a society. I know this from personal experience and I am a white, straight-sized cis woman – from speaking to others who live in bodies that are different to mine and who feel even further from this ideal I have learnt about how much worse this experience can be. Because the 'ideal' is totally unattainable for the vast majority of people – in fact, only around 5 per cent[11] of women *actually* possess the body type typically shown in the media. How does that leave the other 95 per cent of people feeling? Like we don't measure up; like we're not enough. It cultivates body dissatisfaction, which is the experience of negative thoughts and esteem about one's body. Body dissatisfaction has been linked to a range of physical and mental health problems, including disordered eating, body dysmorphic disorder, depression and low self-esteem. It can also be responsible for encouraging body-changing behaviours such as cosmetic surgery, dieting or the use of weight-loss products.

Which is, of course, where diet culture steps in and professes to save the day – it has a solution! Sick of feeling inadequate? Here's our fix! And here's our price . . .

When it's mapped out, it's easy to see how we fall for it, isn't it? Yet another contributing factor is that it catches us at a particularly vulnerable time. During puberty, children gain 50 per cent of their adult body weight,[12] which is, unfortunately, around the same time that people start to become acutely aware of standards and expectations around physical appearance.

There was a fascinating study led by psychiatrist Anne E. Becker in the 1990s that explored body image among young girls. The three-year study measured the effect of television in Fiji, a country with a culture that revolves around food, along with an appreciation for 'large, robust bodies' that was, of course, at odds with the Western ideal. Becker visited Fiji in 1995, a few weeks after television was introduced to the island, and returned in 1998, three years later. Each time, they asked Fijian girls of average age 17 about how much TV they watched, along with questions about their eating behaviours and body image.

The results? Girls who watched TV at least three nights per week were 50 per cent more likely to see themselves as fat (which they viewed in a negative light) and 30 per cent more likely to diet. Risks for developing eating disorders increased significantly – high scores on an eating disorder scale called EAT-26, a screening measure to help determine the presence of an eating disorder, increased 12.7 per cent and induced vomiting to control weight increased 11.3 per cent. Becker concluded that 'key indicators of disordered eating were significantly more prevalent following exposure to television.'

This increase in body dissatisfaction and disordered eating patterns is thought to be down to this new Western, thin body ideal being introduced via TV. Becker quoted from the 1998 interviews: 'I want their body,' said one Fijian girl of the Western shows she watched. 'I want their size.'

These results are frightening when we consider our own level of TV-watching – in the UK, we watch on average over 22.5 hours of TV every week, NOT including streaming services such as Netflix. Which brings me back to the staggering lack of body diversity and representation in film and television. It is very, very rare that we see a person in a larger body on screen. And if we do, their character is being made fun of; they are the butt of the joke and portrayed as gluttonous, dirty, unhygienic, lazy, greedy and even evil.

Let's take the iconic TV show *Friends* and the 'Fat Monica' character, played by Courteney Cox in a fat suit, as an example. When Fat Monica appears on the show, she's either playing into fat stereotypes like constantly eating and crushing objects because of her size or being portrayed as a laughable, unlovable character whose only hope is to lose weight.

The jokes are at her expense and the audience laughs *at* her, not *with* her. Fat Monica has a crush on Chandler and she overhears him making fun of her and being appalled by her weight. It isn't until Fat Monica loses weight the following year as 'revenge' that Chandler is finally able to see an attractive woman and her friends begin to take her seriously.

But this blatant fatphobia is not just seen in *Friends* – remember *Mean Girls*, when Regina George is no longer seen as attractive after gaining weight from eating calorie-dense bars? And in the movie *Sex and the City*, there's a particularly shocking scene where Samantha arrives for Charlotte's baby shower and the group is horrified about her 'weight gain' – genuinely, there is no weight gain to see but it becomes a major talking point among the group. Not to mention TV show *This Is Us*, which gave us a plus-size character with all of the familiar trappings: constant feelings of inadequacy in comparison to the thinner people in her life and engaged in a perpetual battle to lose weight. Her character arc revolves around calories and weight loss. Actress Chrissy Metz excels in the role given to her in the series – her performance earned her a Screen Actors Guild Award for Outstanding Performance – but she deserves way better than the typical 'fat girl' storyline.

Undeniably worse is the depiction of villains in the media as fat, with Disney being one of the worst offenders – particularly troubling when Disney films are the among the first movies young children are likely to watch. Think of characters like Ursula (*The Little Mermaid*), the Queen of Hearts (*Alice in Wonderland*), Madam Min (*The Sword in the Stone*), Governor

The sharp dichotomy laid bare in these Disney films, where evil, feared villains are fat and the loveable heroines are thin, serves to reinforce to young girls the notion that you have to be thin to be beautiful, to be loved and even to be a good person.

Ratcliffe (*Pocahontas*), Lawrence (*The Princess and the Frog*) and Pete (*Mickey Mouse universe*) – all villains, all fat, with common traits in these characters including selfishness, greed and cruelty. These are, in turn, the associations that children are taught to make about fat people.

Another Disney example is the matchmaker from the film *Mulan*, a fat woman who is responsible for arranging marriages and evaluating potential brides and grooms. Yet she doesn't have a partner herself – it is merely her job to teach all of the thin women how to be good wives. Which brings us to another problem – the contrast of these fat characters with the thin, beautiful women who play the heroines. There is an absolute lack of full-bodied – or even average-sized – protagonists in Disney movies. Think about it: Cinderella, Snow White, Pocahontas, Belle, Jasmine, Ariel: all impossibly thin, yet with a perfect hourglass figure. It is, therefore, no surprise that when Professor Hayes and Professor Tantleff-Dunn asked girls under the age of six to select the 'real princess' from a choice of ballerinas, as part of their 2009 experiment, 50 per cent chose the thinnest one. A third of those girls also admitted to worrying about being fat.[13]

The sharp dichotomy laid bare in these Disney films, where evil, feared villains are fat and the lovable heroines are thin, serves to reinforce to young girls the notion that you have to be thin to be beautiful, to be loved and even to be a good person. The harm caused is crystal clear.

But the harm doesn't only lie with fictional films and TV series. It's difficult to discuss media portrayal of fat people without mentioning reality shows like *The Biggest Loser* and *Supersize vs. Superskinny*. *The Biggest Loser* was an incredibly successful US television show that took advantage of people desperate to lose weight – the contestants were subjected to extreme dieting and gruelling exercise in a bid to become the 'Biggest Loser'. The show greatly contributed to a common – and very harmful – misconception that fatness is caused solely by individual failure rather than a mixture of complex factors including environment and genes.

*Supersize vs. Superskinny*, on the other hand, was a UK show that saw a fat person swap their diet with a thin person (yep, I'm not getting the logic there, either). The pair were brought to a feeding clinic, where a number of ridiculous rituals, including each contestant's weekly food intake slopped into a giant plastic tube in order to evoke feelings of shame and disgust, were carried out. They then lived together for five days, during which viewers would gawp as the thin person attempted to force down takeaways and the fat person lived on morsels of food. It was an utterly horrendous and seriously triggering premise but it made for incredibly compulsive viewing – especially for those with an eating disorder, myself included. It was my favourite

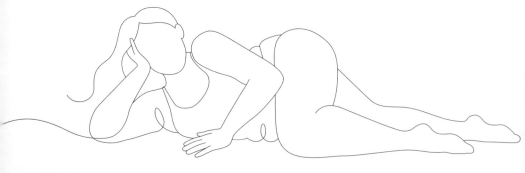

show on TV for a long time, I'm embarrassed to admit. I had a ritual – I needed to watch it alone, with my dinner. But watching it would prevent me from eating my dinner: the talks of weight, calories, eating habits and the level of disgust aimed at the fat person meant that I was only able to manage a few mouthfuls. And, given the mental state I was in at that time, that felt to me like a good thing. So, week after week, I continued to watch it, along with a huge portion of the eating disorder community, until it was cancelled in 2014 after a six-year run.

Essentially, TV and film have normalised bullying fat people and largely contributed to and perpetuated the notion that fat people are bad and thin people are good. When we see fat people on TV, they're either ridiculed, pitied, the villain or they're performing for the viewers as a 'good fatty' – this is a term I've often heard on social media, coined by fat people, to describe a fat person trying to lose weight. They are deemed 'good' because this character has recognised that their body is unacceptable and they are trying to do the 'right thing' and correct that.

When larger-bodied actors do appear on our screens, they are rarely, if ever, afforded nuance in their roles or a complex character arc, like their slimmer-bodied colleagues. But in reality, we hardly ever see them, as the lack of representation of fat people has meant that we are practically brainwashed to believe that they don't belong in the media. So when there is a body on screen that differs from the typical slim woman, it comes as a shock.

I remember watching the HBO series *Girls*, which first came out in 2012, and being stunned that the protagonist, Hannah

Horvath, played by Lena Dunham, wasn't thin. She also wasn't fat, but for television, she was big – and she wasn't allowed to forget this, being subjected to constant fat-shaming in the press. She told the *Guardian*, 'My fears came true: people called me fat and hideous.' Joan Rivers famously referenced Lena's weight in a radio interview, saying that it sent the wrong message to girls. 'She's sending a message out to people that it's OK to stay fat and get diabetes,' she said. 'I'm saying if you like the way you look, Lena, that's fine, and you're funny, but don't say it's OK that other girls look like this. Tell them to try and look better.' Speaking of Lena's fashion sense, she even went on to ask, 'How could she wear dresses above the knee?' Why – because she's not thin?! Gross.

This seems to be a good time to touch on fat men in film and TV: while the same stereotypes are applied as to women, these characters are more readily afforded nuance and complexity. They are more likely to have storylines unrelated to weight and/or be shown in a positive, more appealing or affectionate light than fat women – think Homer Simpson, Patrick Star from *SpongeBob SquarePants*, Philip Banks from *The Fresh Prince of Bel-Air*, Dan Conner from *Roseanne*, Fred Flintstone and Cameron Tucker from *Modern Family*. All characters whose storylines don't consistently revolve around their weight.

When I was a young teenager, social media really only stretched to MSN messenger and MySpace, available on my desktop computer via dial-up internet. My early impressions of the thin, successful woman I was supposed to aspire to be came from TV, film, advertising and magazines. Now, courtesy of social media and the smartphones that we keep within reach pretty much 24 hours a day, it's entirely possible, or even quite likely, to feel caught in a constant flow of images of the 'perfect' body, like a tap you can't turn off.

Social media is, of course, a wonderful thing in many ways but we're still finding out about some of the consequences of the negative effects it can have on us. As I was writing this chapter, news leaked that Facebook has kept internal research secret for two years that suggests its app, Instagram, makes body image issues worse for teenage girls. And that they have failed to do anything about it. A leaked slide from an internal presentation given in 2019, seen by *The Wall Street Journal*, reads: 'We make body image issues worse for one in three teen girls.' A subsequent presentation reportedly from March 2020 said: 'Thirty-two per cent of teen girls said that when they felt bad about their bodies, Instagram made them feel worse.'

What makes this news even more insidious is that Instagram algorithms push teenage girls who even briefly engage with fitness-related images towards a flood of weight-loss content, according to research carried out by people attempting to recreate the experience of being a child on social networks. One account that was set up in the name of a 17-year-old girl liked one single post from a sportswear brand about dieting that appeared on her 'explore' tab and followed an account that was suggested to her after it posted a 'before and after' weight-loss journey photo. These two actions alone were sufficient for the algorithm to steer her towards this content and the researchers found her explore feed suddenly began to feature substantially more content relating to weight-loss stories and tips, fitness content and body sculpting. The content often featured 'noticeably slim, and in some cases seemingly edited/distorted body shapes.'[14] The experiment was carried out several more times in similar circumstances with similar results. Scary, right? We talk about social media in more depth in Chapter 13.

As I continue to write, I'm becoming increasingly aware of how negative this chapter is, which is pretty unavoidable given that we're talking about the media and its effect on our collective body image and self-esteem. But I want to leave you with some positivity because things *are* getting better and we *are* taking steps in the right direction, even if progress is slow and the social media giants appear to be doing nothing to help.

The media industry is, on the whole, becoming progressively more inclusive, with women of lots of different shapes and sizes gracing billboards, magazine covers, television and catwalks. Rihanna's lingerie line, Savage X Fenty, was widely praised for its diverse line-up when it debuted at New York Fashion Week in 2018, while plus-size model Tess Holliday stormed the runway for Chromat in 2020. *Vogue* featured plus-size model Ashley Graham on its cover in 2017 – their first ever plus-size cover – but the historically famously fatphobic fashion bible really broke new ground when they featured fat superstar singer Lizzo on their October 2020 cover.

Victoria's Secret, the lingerie brand famous for their catwalk bonanza displaying their ultra-thin gaggle of 'angels' was forced to cancel their fashion show in 2019, stating the concept needed to be redefined 'in a way that's culturally relevant' amid controversy over transphobia, a lack of inclusivity and diversity and low viewing figures. In 2021, they announced their plan to 'rebrand', overhauling their image with a more inclusive message.

*Don't get me wrong – it's far from perfect.*

Many of the plus-size models that are used to provide diversity in campaigns are still often women with an hourglass figure and a flat stomach and possibly not above a UK size 14/16. The most famous plus-size models are also still predominantly white – a sign of the systemic racism that exists in the fashion industry. So, yeah, there's still a lot of work to be done, but I am hopeful this is providing a sort of 'gateway' into true diversity and representation.

Television and film still have a really long way to go, we cannot deny that, but hopefully the release of series like *Shrill*, where the protagonist is a fat woman whose focus lies outside of changing her body, and its positive audience response, is a sign of the industry heading in the right direction.

Call me naive but I think we're getting somewhere. There are, however, some barriers we need to break down first . . .

# CHAPTER 4

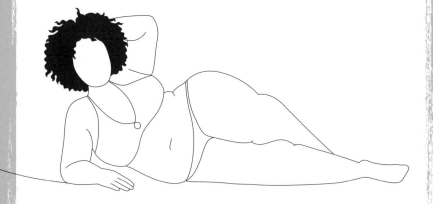

# Weight

# ≠ health

The belief that you can only be healthy if you are thin is so deeply ingrained that it often goes completely unquestioned.

Even by the medical establishment.

If you are fat then you must be unhealthy. This belief has helped the diet industry to flourish. Not only have we been told our bodies must look a certain way to be acceptable but if they don't, we are running a high risk of all sorts of health conditions. Gyms, weight-loss products, liposuction and gastric bypass surgeries all rely heavily on the message that being 'overweight' is highly detrimental to your health.

In order to dismantle diet culture, we need to readdress how our society looks at health and wellness. Equating weight with health perpetuates diet culture and helps maintain the thin ideal. It also reinforces fatphobia (more on this in the next chapter), weight stigma and contributes to keeping people locked in a cycle of causing devastating damage to their bodies. It means that health professionals misdiagnose people in larger bodies – so all pervasive is the assumption that you are unhealthy if you are fat that it can blind doctors to real health problems.

So we *have* to separate out the two, to bust the myth that fat bodies are always unhealthy bodies. Because, despite everything you have been told, it's not true. This is, clearly, a huge topic that we're not going to be able to solve in one chapter but let's aim to tackle some of our existing beliefs around weight and health, with the guidance of a medical doctor.

First of all, let's talk about what 'healthy' even means, which in itself is pretty complex, so buckle in! As far back as 1948, the World Health Organization (WHO) defined health as 'a state of complete physical, mental, and social wellbeing and not merely the absence of disease or infirmity'. In 1986, they made further clarifications: 'A resource for everyday life, not the objective of living. Health is a positive concept emphasising social and personal resources, as well as physical capacities.' Essentially, health is a resource to support our function in wider society, rather than the goal itself.

Here are some other definitions of health you will find being used by experts:

- An absence of disease.

- A state that allows an individual to adequately cope with the demands of daily life.

- A state of balance that an individual has established within himself and between himself and his social and physical environment.[15]

But from my research, talking to experts and thinking about it a lot, I believe that a significant amount of the meaning lies in context and circumstance. Health is nuanced, it encompasses a variety of different factors – including nutritional intake, exercise, stress, mental health, social health and financial health – and looks different for different people.

But while the term is a little muddy, one thing is crystal clear: you cannot see health. You cannot look at a person and know whether or not they're in good health. You know nothing about their eating patterns, their nutritional intake, their exercise regime, their stress levels, their sleep health, the state of their mental health or any other health-related behaviour from the way they appear.

'Health is totally person and context-dependant,' says NHS doctor, nutritionist and author of *Food Isn't Medicine* Joshua Wolrich. 'And it's actually important not to have a concrete definition of health in our head because it can change. It also might be something we have no capacity to ever achieve because the vast majority of factors are way beyond our control.' Such factors include genetics, oppression, environmental factors and socioeconomic status: while inequality exists, says Wolrich, it is almost impossible to find a one-size-fits-all definition for health.

## OK, so we can't say exactly what it means to be healthy. Can we define who is fat?

The tool most used in medicine to screen for weight categories is BMI – body mass index, which is calculated by dividing your weight by the square of your body height. I think BMI is one of the things that crops up most in my DMs. I get lots of messages from women who consider themselves very healthy, visit their doctors and are told they are in the wrong BMI bracket and need to lose weight. We are relentlessly taught to fear fat, to fear being 'overweight', so then, when we find out that our BMI puts us in that category, or even defines us as 'obese' or 'morbidly obese', it can feel deeply unpleasant.

We'll get onto why that's so problematic in a minute but for now, let's dive into what the BMI is and where it came from.

Adolphe Quetelet was a Belgian academic interested in studying human traits in relation to mortality. He studied astronomy, mathematics, statistics and sociology, but was not a doctor, physician or expert in health. Driven to find *l'homme moyen* (the average man) in 1830 (yes, nearly 200 years ago) he devised the Quetelet Index. He derived the index from a simple maths formula involving a weight-to-height ratio, which was based on the size and measurements collected from white French and Scottish participants. Quetelet explicitly said that the index was designed for use on a population level, NOT an individual level. In other words, it was supposed to be used to give us stats about the physical traits of people in general, not to assess any one person.

At this time, weight wasn't considered to be one of the principal factors contributing to health. However, in the early twentieth century, health insurance companies began linking 'excessive' body fat with an increased risk of heart disease.[16] Life insurances companies in the US decided to devise weight and height tables in order to determine what to charge policyholders. Insurers could then refuse to cover the 'overweight' patients or charge them more. The method was clearly flawed and produced inconsistent results but it remained in place and, soon, physicians adopted these rating tables to assess the weight and, therefore, health, of their patients, with many doctors refusing to take on patients in higher weight categories.

In the 1970s, amid a growing dissatisfaction with the unreliability of the tables, researcher Ancel Keys (who conducted the 1944 Minnesota Starvation Experiment, and who we met in Chapter two) claimed to have a more accurate tool to measure body fat – the Quetelet Index. He and a group of fellow researchers carried out a study of 7,500 men from five different countries – the US, Italy, Finland, Japan and South Africa. They concluded that, despite being less than 'satisfactory', Quetelet's body mass index (measuring weight against height) was the most reliable way of measuring body fat – of various different tested methods. So, they weren't even saying it was a really good system, it was just the most reliable of the ones they tried (which included immersing someone in water followed by a seven-minute nitrogen washout to approximate lung volume for the body density calculation and measuring the volume of gastrointestinal gases). Phew – that was a mouthful!

The study renamed Quetelet's Index the 'Body Mass Index' and in 1985, the method was officially approved for medical use in the US. There were just two categories then – healthy and overweight. Men with a BMI score over 27.8 and women over 27.3 were to be deemed overweight and therefore unhealthy.

But in 1998, the National Institutes of Health lowered the 'overweight' threshold from 27.8 and 27.3 to 25 and added a new 'obese' category for anything over 30. This change made roughly 29 million Americans 'unhealthy' overnight[17] and critics claimed that the new guidelines were drafted partly by the International Obesity Task Force, whose two main funders were companies selling weight-loss drugs. In 1997, the same task force expanded the number of BMI categories to include different degrees of 'obesity'. The arbitrary and contrived nature of these distinctions are becoming quite clear, are they not?

Today, the BMI is as follows: if you're below 18.5, you're underweight; 18.5–24.9 is normal; 25–29.9 is overweight; 30–40 is obese and anything over 40 is morbidly obese.

I'm sure you've figured most of these out for yourself by now but let's quickly look at some of the rather glaring flaws in the BMI scale and at what happens when you apply this basic tool to real people.

Firstly, the Quetelet Index and the ensuing Body Mass Index were both based on measuring white men. Body mass varies across different ethnicities and so anyone who falls outside of these male, European standards is not represented. This is illustrated by statistics that show Black people are more likely to fall into higher BMI categories than other ethnic groups. While, in fact, higher or lower BMIs might be healthier for different groups of people. For Black people, for example, a higher BMI tends to be more optimal.[18] Yet the same BMI method is applied globally, regardless of ethnicity or gender.

Secondly, BMI was never intended for use on an individual level. 'Whenever we put something into categories, we're always going to create problems when we try to apply that individually,' says Dr Wolrich. 'Categories are fine at a population level but not on an individual level.' There is, of course, a difference between having oversight of a population's average statistics and using the categories to implement health measures at an individual level.

BMI was never
intended for use on
an individual level.

BMI doesn't just skip over important details around ethnicity, it fails to take into account questions of body composition – such as bone density, fat distribution and muscle. This lack of differentiation between muscle and fat is the reason why athletes often fall into the higher categories – the average male rugby forward playing in Europe, for example, is 1.9m tall and weighs 112.5kg, which put them into the 'obese' category.[19] The bottom line is that a BMI result simply cannot automatically deem someone healthy or unhealthy.

Another thing that BMI doesn't account for is age. In fact, a 2013 analysis looked at 97 studies covering nearly 3 million people and determined that those in the overweight bracket were 6 per cent less likely to die in a given year than those in the normal range, with this percentage even higher for middle-aged and elderly people.[20] 'The World Health Organization calls BMIs of 25 to 29.9 overweight,' said Paul McAuley, an exercise researcher at Winston-Salem State University. 'That is actually what is healthiest for middle-aged Americans.' Furthermore, people with high BMIs tend to have a history of dieting, which is known to have a negative effect on health. 'So does illness come from having a higher BMI or from inflammation in the blood due to dieting?' Bacon asked. 'We just don't know.'

I find it so unbelievable that such an arbitrary, inaccurate method – it is, essentially, a 200-year-old hack that was never invented with health in mind – is so universally relied on to determine someone's health. And that it has been for so long without being properly challenged. I guess that's testament to our nature as humans to blindly adopt and obey systems of authority:

the BMI is ingrained in our medical systems and has been for so long that it's just part and parcel of today's healthcare.

And, unfortunately, it can have serious consequences: if BMI is deemed too high, patients can be denied IVF, surgeries and certain medications. It's used as a tool to discriminate. It's very, very common for someone to visit their doctor, get weighed, be placed into a higher than 'normal' BMI category and be told to lose weight. I know that because of the aforementioned amount of DMs I receive that detail this very situation. Patients are encouraged to diet – you know: 'eat less, move more!' – which is *so* toxic when you consider the implications of intentional weight loss . . .

We've seen how dieting almost never works: initial weight loss may occur but it almost always ends in weight gain. What 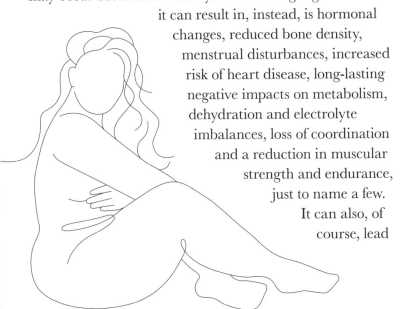 it can result in, instead, is hormonal changes, reduced bone density, menstrual disturbances, increased risk of heart disease, long-lasting negative impacts on metabolism, dehydration and electrolyte imbalances, loss of coordination and a reduction in muscular strength and endurance, just to name a few. It can also, of course, lead to a dysfunctional relationship with food and even an eating disorder. So while your doctor believes that encouraging you to lose weight will improve your health, if you follow their advice, you're actually more likely to worsen your health. Crazy, right?

I experienced this when I visited my GP at the age of 18, shortly after starting university, for what I thought was depression. I was homesick, miserable away from my family and struggling to cope with being on my own for the first time ever, and desperately wanted help. The doctor I saw was a man roughly in his sixties who immediately told me to get on the scales. I obliged, of course. My BMI number fell into the 'obese' category and I was told I needed to lose weight. I left the doctor's feeling just as low, except now I had the added anxiety of believing that I needed to lose weight – and fast. This experience prompted me to sign up to a Slimming World class in my new city and I went on to lose a stone in a matter of weeks. I gained it back – and a bit more – pretty swiftly after. So, of course, I moved on to another diet. I know this is an experience that will resonate with many of you.

What I didn't know, back then – and, truthfully, I actually didn't know this until very recently – is that you can say 'no' to being weighed at the doctors. This sounds so simple when I type it out – like, of course you can! – but it's something that just didn't occur to me; I just thought we *had* to. Again, back to us blindly obeying authority.

'You are absolutely in charge,' says Dr Wolrich. 'I think it's important to ask the doctor why they want to weigh you. If it's to do with calculating dosage for a medication or checking on an unexplained weight fluctuation (weight loss is often one of the first signs of cancer) then yes, it's important. But if it's just to update the system or check on your BMI, you can say no. Whether you get weighed or not is in your hands, but asking why, as a patient, is really important – especially if you want to be involved in your health. We need to question more.'

I should have asked my doctor why he wanted to weigh me when I was visiting for low mood. In fact, I should have just said 'no': my weight had nothing to do with my current mental state.

If you do get weighed and you are told to lose weight, ask your doctor what the reason is. Get to the root of *why* they are asking you to lose weight – and don't be scared to point them towards resources that illustrate either the inefficacy of intentional weight loss and/or the statistics about weight and its relations to health. This weight-centred approach to health needs to change – because being stigmatised for your weight can be a bigger risk to your health than what you eat or what you weigh – but in order for that to happen, it needs to be challenged.

Pinning health on weight is not only totally reductive – it is dangerous. We'll talk more about this in the next chapter, as this is clear fatphobia, but the reality is that when a fat person visits the doctor, they can find that their health concerns are dismissed out of hand, they are prescribed weight loss for unrelated illnesses or even that they get misdiagnosed. These mistakes mean that fat people are less likely to visit their doctors and potential illnesses are picked up later than they could have been.

Being stigmatised for your weight can be a bigger risk to your health than what you eat or what you weigh.

'Healthcare tends to take a "weight-normative" approach, with an overarching focus on weight and weight loss as a means to health, and this results in discrimination of those who don't fit within its narrow definition,' says Dr Wolrich. It also means that fat people who have eating disorders are far less likely to get diagnosed because they don't fit the typical stereotype of someone with an eating disorder: a very thin girl . . . Because NEWSFLASH:

*You can't see an eating disorder.*

Our assumptions about size and health don't just disadvantage fat people: when people with 'normal' BMIs are automatically assumed to be healthy, things like their nutrition, sleep, stress and movement, for example, are left unquestioned. That person, however, may well be battling disordered eating, an eating disorder or a physical illness that goes undiagnosed.

The assumptions are also just plain wrong: 'It is absolutely possible for someone who falls in the "obese" bracket on the BMI scale to be completely medically healthy,' says Dr Wolrich. 'It's also possible for someone who falls into the "healthy" bracket on the BMI scale to be medically unhealthy.'

While it's true that both low weights and high weights *can* have a negative impact on your health, it is nowhere near as clear-cut or straightforward as we're led to believe. Dr Wolrich explains: 'It depends on where in the body the fat is stored – evidence suggests that increasing visceral fat [found deep below the skin, around your vital organs] has the biggest potential harmful impact on our health, followed by subcutaneous fat [more visible fat just under the skin] around the abdomen. But research also shows that increased subcutaneous fat in the hips and thighs is actually protective for metabolic health in adults of all ages. Higher levels of body fat in postmenopausal women is also protective against both osteoporosis and the mortality associated with fragility fractures.

'Prior to menopause, lower levels of fat can have negative impacts on hormone production and can even lead to a condition where periods stop for a certain period of time – this has been linked to an increased risk of cardiovascular disease and reduced bone density. Not to mention that body fat can also be protective when we get sick: fat patients are more likely to survive admission to an intensive care unit when unwell.'

So, without really getting into the weeds (I'll leave that to the experts – I recommend Dr Wolrich's book for further reading): yes, carrying too much fat *can* impact someone's health. But it's something that should be explored and determined on a case-by-case basis, not just by looking at someone or putting them into a certain BMI category.

'Fat is neither healthy nor unhealthy,' wrote Fall Ferguson, JD, MA, in a blog piece for the Association for Size Diversity and Health (ASDAH). 'Being fat has been correlated with some health conditions, but its role in causing disease is highly exaggerated. What the data do clearly show is that many people are both fat and healthy. Moreover, merely removing adipose tissue via liposuction has no effect on health whatsoever. This all suggests that we need to look for other causes than adipose tissue for the health conditions that tend to be blamed on "obesity".'

*To summarise: weight does not determine health.*

So what's the alternative? A movement that is, fortunately, growing in popularity: Health at Every Size (HAES). HAES, which originated in the 1960s, is a means to address weight bias and stigma against fat individuals, recognising that fat people often compromise their health in persistent attempts to lose weight. 'HAES is a framework that, at its core, believes that every person has the right to pursue health habits without the measure from the scale,' says HAES body image coach and educator Brianna M. Campos (@bodyimagewithbri). 'HAES is inherently a social justice issue. It argues that health is beyond body size, but also social factors, socioeconomic factors and income disparities.'

According to the Association for Size Diversity and Health (ASDAH), HAES promotes:

- **Weight inclusivity**, by acknowledging and respecting the inherent diversity of body shapes and sizes and rejecting the idealising or pathologising of specific weights.

- **Health enhancement**, by supporting health policies that improve and equalise access to information and services.

- **Eating for wellbeing**, by promoting flexible, individualised eating based on hunger, satiety, nutritional needs and pleasure, rather than externally regulated eating focused on weight control.

- **Respectful care**, by acknowledging biases and working to end weight discrimination, weight stigma and weight bias.

- **Life-enhancing movement**, by supporting physical activities that allow people of all sizes, abilities and interests to engage in enjoyable movement.

Dr Wolrich uses a HAES approach with his patients: 'To have an approach that is weight-inclusive, where we are looking at things where success isn't judged by how much weight is lost, is very important. Judging exercise, for example, on whether it has been successful in regard to the number on the scales is incredibly problematic. Not only is it simply nonsense (exercise *always* improves our health), as soon as the number stops changing, we stop exercising. 'As doctors we're meant to be promoting health, yet by encouraging its conflation with weight we're doing our patients a huge disservice. Far more of us need to be reading and learning about HAES and not just rejecting it because people are calling it "healthy at every size".'

The only difference is a 'y' but it's a big distinction: HAES doesn't deem people healthy at every size – that's impossible to claim – it is simply promoting a *focus* on health at every size, regardless of weight. It doesn't mean denying the impact that lots of things can have on health, but it does mean understanding that a subject so complicated, nuanced and context-dependent as health requires a similar approach.

As it stands, our healthcare systems still have a long way to go when it comes to banishing the BMI scale and adopting HAES, but I asked Dr Wolrich how he envisaged health outcomes if both were to disappear overnight. 'The general health of the population would increase; I have no doubt about that. At the moment, we have swathes of the population who believe the only way they can improve their health is to lose weight and they are obsessed with weight loss as a goal, which means that people are missing out on health-promoting behaviours that they have the capacity for and ability for,' he says.

Referring to weight stigma and medical discrimination against fat people, he says: 'It would allow a lot of people – who are currently refusing to because of previous poor treatment – to come back to seeing their healthcare providers

Health is not a
look or size.

If someone assumes
your health based on
how you look, it's their
mindset that needs
addressing, not your
body size.

and trust in them to help improve or maintain their health.'

So, how can we start to shift the way we view our own health away from weight and towards other factors that influence our wellbeing?

I've thought long and hard about what 'healthy' means for me while writing this chapter. And I've come to the conclusion that a huge part of health is actually nothing to do with my physical body, rather my mental wellbeing. Am I managing my anxiety? Am I allowing myself enough rest? Am I keeping my stress levels low? Of course, it comprises other factors, too, like whether I'm eating enough fruit and veg, getting enough sleep and moving my body on a semi-regular basis, but it starts with my mind. Don't get me wrong: I don't think mental health is, in general, more important than physical health, but for me, it's important that I prioritise my mental health. That way, my physical health largely follows.

For someone else, it might be a focus on sleep health, or their interpersonal relationships – it's so individual that I can't tell you what 'health' should mean and be for you; I think that's something that will be beneficial for you to explore – with weight firmly out of the picture.

But no matter what you land on, please know that health is not a look or size. And if someone assumes your health based on how you look, it's their mindset that needs addressing, not your body size.

# CHAPTER 5

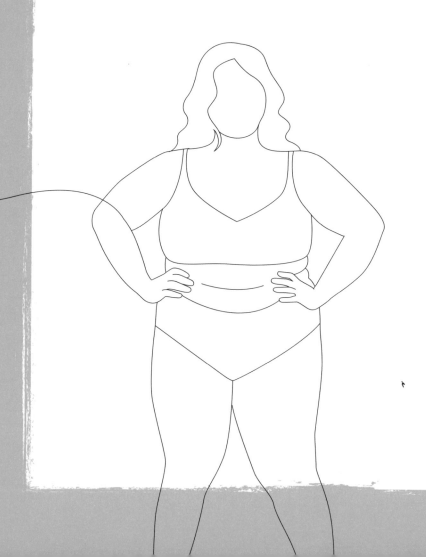

'Fat' is not
a bad word

# Fatphobia, if you're not familiar with the term, is the fear and hatred of fat bodies.

It is a form of discrimination that equates fatness with inferiority, undesirability and immorality and results in a plethora of damaging mental and physical consequences for fat people.

And yet, in many ways, it remains a socially acceptable form of discrimination – fat people are still the butt of the jokes in film and television, as well as in comedians' routines, and casually mocked in the street.

According to one 2018 survey, more than four in five UK adults believe fat people are viewed negatively because of their weight and 62 per cent of Brits think people are likely to discriminate against someone who is fat.[21] The findings also showed that fat people experience stigma and discrimination across all aspects of their lives: nearly half of adults who are fat have felt judged because of their weight in clothes shops or in social situations and, even more concerningly, in healthcare settings (45 per cent) and gyms (32 per cent).

Fatphobia lies at the very heart of diet culture, so, in order to take it down, we have to dismantle fatphobia. If you're not fat, you might be surprised at just how ubiquitous – and overt – fatphobia is. Instances include: doctors refusing to treat fat people properly and attributing every medical problem to their body size; unsolicited body shaming and/or weight loss advice from strangers; the depiction of onscreen fat characters, as we discussed in Chapter four, as lazy, unintelligent or unattractive; aggression on public transport – especially planes due to the size of the seats; workplace discrimination; romantic discrimination; clothing brands refusing to cater for bigger bodies and even lower wages – one US study found that fat women were predicted almost $10,000 less in salary than thin women and larger fat people a staggering $19,000 less.[22] Fatphobia causes untold damage and is a huge concern – and not just for fat people. In order to truly dismantle it, those of us who aren't fat need to speak up and advocate against it, too. In an ideal world, fat people would be listened to about their experiences and what they think is best for them, but prejudices get in the way. However, the privilege of a thin person means, unfortunately, that their voices are far louder. It's essential that non-marginalised people step up to fight all kinds of oppression: in order to live in a world that is equal for all shapes, sizes, genders, races and abilities, people with privilege must push back against biases and shout the loudest. Because it is in *all* of our interests.

How did you feel about the way I have been using the word 'fat' so far? I know it can be jarring to hear, so why am I using it? Author and content creator Stephanie Yeboah, who is a Black, fat woman, explained to me her take on why it's important that we use this word: 'The word "fat" in the general lexicon has long been used by society as an insult to those who live in larger bodies,' she said. 'Like similar descriptive words such as "slim", "tall", "Black" and "white", fat is a neutral word that exists just to describe the shape of bodies that store extra fat.

'Over the years, I've learnt to reclaim the word in a bid to take back the power and the negativity that society has placed on it. I'm fat because I have extra fat. Fat doesn't make me unworthy, ugly or undesirable. It makes me fat! If we can call ourselves fat, then it cannot be weaponised against us.'

Which makes sense: for those living in a society determined to villainise and marginalise fat people because of an arbitrary beauty standard, reclaiming the word and letting it shed its

'Fat doesn't make me unworthy, ugly or undesirable.'

STEPHANIE YEBOAH

negative connotations is powerful and liberating. 'Fat' is not a pejorative, but an adjective. But should non-fat people use the word to describe body types? I asked Yeboah. 'In order to remove the stigma and the general negativity of the word, I'd encourage non-fat people to routinely use the word, as it can hopefully become more normalised within society. My hope is that down the line, everyone will be able to use it as just a body descriptor and nothing else,' she said.

However, while it's important for us to start normalising the word, we also need to bear in mind that, given the deeply anti-fat world that we live in, a softly-softly approach is key. 'In the current climate, the use of the word "fat" is still met with resistance from fat people who aren't as far along in their self-love journey as others. And it's understandable! It will take a long time to get to a point where we unlearn all of the toxic, negative narratives surrounding that word,' says Yeboah. She advises using the word on a case-by-case basis and making sure that your fat friends feel comfortable with you using the word in front of them or to describe their body shape: it's important they give their consent.

This raises the issue of: how do you know when someone is fat? At what particular point does someone go from being 'non-fat' to 'fat'? Unqualified to answer this myself, I'm going to quote fat activist and author Aubrey Gordon, from an article she wrote for *Medium*: 'Truthfully, there are no clear answers . . . every definition of fat is deeply flawed at worst, relative at best. BMI standards have been manipulated over time, adjusted most notably in 1998, when millions of Americans went to sleep with bodies prized by the BMI as healthy weight, and woke up the disappointing overweight or worse, the reviled obese,' she wrote.

What's more, the definition of fat varies according to country, culture, family and person. 'As a fat person,' Gordon wrote, 'all I can trust is self-identity. If you, in your heart of hearts, know yourself to be fat, then you are . . . I choose to believe people who tell me they're fat. But when I look for my fat people – the community I call home – I think of people who are united by experiences of widespread, inescapable exclusion. Not just people who've been called fat, all of us have, but folks who are shut out from meeting their basic needs because of the simple fact of their size. Not just people who struggle to find clothing they like, but people who struggle to find clothing at all . . . For my fat people, our size isn't just an internal worry, it's an inescapable, external reality.'

I know it's a grey area, and I'm sorry I can't make it more clear, but I believe what's vital is consent from an individual before labelling them a 'fat' person, while still being able to refer to the fat population as a whole as 'fat' and not being fearful of the word.

There are two words, however, that I won't be using in this chapter – 'obesity' and 'overweight'. And I ask that you reconsider your use of them, too. Let's explore why. 'Overweight' is a bit of stupid one that doesn't require much explanation because . . . over *what* weight?! It just quite simply makes no sense.

Originally coined by medical services as a term to discuss potential health risks associated with fatness, 'obesity' is now a word used to stigmatise and discriminate. We've all seen the scaremongering 'obesity epidemic' headlines and yet the term is often used by the government to scapegoat communities and distract from other societal problems like poverty – and it's now commonly used as an insult to fat people. It's also a word whose definition is built on very shaky ground: in medical terms, 'obesity' applies to anyone with a BMI of 30 or higher. And, as we've seen, BMI is . . . pretty dodgy, to put it one way.

## Essentially, 'obesity' and 'overweight' are now entwined with fatphobia.

Of course, this discrimination is heightened when the fat person is marginalised in another area, because of race, gender, sexuality, or disability, for example. Yeboah explains: 'Existing in a body that crosses various intersections (fat, Black, darker-skinned) gives ample opportunity for people to abuse, police and discriminate against my body. Fat Black women have to navigate this world a lot differently than fat white women, as fat white women still have the privilege of being white, which will always be a standard of beauty. Not only that, but white women are afforded a grace, leniency and a sense of innocence that Black women are never given.'

Writing about fatphobia is definitely one of the hardest topics in this book for me to tackle because I am attempting to describe and explain a form of discrimination that I have never been subject to. Yes, I don't look quite like the typical model you tend to see on advertisements but I benefit from thin privilege and my body is socially accepted. Layer on top the fact that I am white; I don't and have never faced systemic oppression for how my body looks.

Thin privilege means, according to anti-diet activist and registered dietitian Christy Harrison, 'that by virtue of some characteristic of your body – in this case, being below a certain size – you have greater access to resources and face less discrimination in society than people without that characteristic.'

When I speak about thin privilege on Instagram, I'm often met with a lot of confusion: 'How can I be privileged if I don't feel thin?' or 'How can I be privileged if I hate my body?' The answer is that you don't have to feel thin or not hate your body to have thin privilege – thinness isn't a feeling, it's an actual body type. It's how you are viewed and treated by the outside world. You might not feel thin but that doesn't mean that you suffer from discrimination because of your body size. You might not like your body but you are still able to navigate the world without the added stress of having to worry about not being able to buy clothes or fit into aeroplane seats. You are still able to eat in public without worrying about being shamed.

When I was in the depths of my eating disorder and living in a body I almost physically couldn't bear, I still had thin privilege. My inner negativity about myself was not *also* reflected back at me by society.

There's also the question of 'Well, how can I have thin privilege if people shame me for my thin body?' Of course, people of all shapes and sizes receive comments about how they look – and thin people are often on the receiving end of comments such as

Body shaming
is NEVER OK –
no matter what
shape or size
you are.

'Eat a burger!' or 'Real women have curves' (a particularly gross term because all women are real) – and that is never acceptable. Body shaming is NEVER OK – no matter what shape or size you are. But thin-shaming is not the same as the systemic and overwhelming bias that we know exists against fat bodies and I believe we can all acknowledge that difference without letting it take away from any of the things that we suffer from.

Fatphobia is rife and shows up in many different ways; it is engrained in Western culture and, often, we aren't even aware of it. Stephanie Yeboah details some of her experiences with weight bias: 'As a larger-fat person (a UK size 24), I have had several experiences with fatphobia which have mostly shown up within healthcare, dating and generally being out and about in public. 'I have had experiences going to the GP to talk about skin/bruising issues, only for the GP to take one look at my body and invite me to hop on the scale, citing my weight as the reason for the bruising. I've also had my weight listed as the reason for having asthma, despite my slim father and brother also having the disease (it is actually something I inherited). It doesn't make me feel like my health concerns are treated with any kind of care or degree of seriousness, which in the long term could prove fatal if I were to have a serious illness that went untreated because of the assumption of my weight being the issue.'

This aspect of fatphobia is particularly troubling, as weight stigma is a dangerous threat to health – and it is not limited to psychological distress and physical illness, it also extends to risk of mortality.[23] This may be for several reasons: as Stephanie illustrated, doctors often refuse to look past weight to treat physical health, which can lead to lapses in treatment;

the healthcare system is often ill-prepared for fat people as it is designed for thin people, with machines for diagnostic purposes like CT and MRI scanners not having been built big enough; surgeons often refuse to operate on fat people; drug doses are usually based on thin body sizes and fat people are less likely to go to the doctors until absolutely necessary because of the weight stigma they face. In cancer, for example, fat patients are thought to have worse outcomes and a higher risk of death, according to Dr Clifford Hudis, chief executive of the American Society of Clinical Oncology.

The dangers of weight stigma hit the mainstream recently after an American woman called Amanda Lee, 27, took to TikTok to detail her experience with the medical system. Amanda had been suffering with abdominal cramps for months, to the point where it was impacting her daily functioning and eating habits. When she described to her physician that the pain was preventing her from eating, he replied: 'Maybe that isn't such a bad thing.' The doctor declined to run any tests on Amanda and she left with a prescription for a urinary tract infection (which she didn't have). In the car after the appointment, Amanda cried as she explained her experience and the video went viral. Spurred on to get a second opinion, Amanda visited a female doctor and immediately underwent a colonoscopy – a large tumour was found in her colon and she was diagnosed with stage three cancer. There are, unfortunately, many more similar stories and they go to show how dangerous and life-threatening weight stigma continues to be.

For Stephanie Yeboah, being a victim of fatphobia

understandably had great impact on her mental and physical health: 'It took a toll on me in my early twenties, which resulted in me experimenting with an array of different dieting programmes, as well as fasting. I put my body through hell and I became ill due to extreme weight loss. My self-esteem was incredibly low, as I didn't deem myself worth enough to be loved, desired or wanted.'

Romantic life has also been problematic for Yeboah as a plus-size woman: 'With dating, I have been in several situations where despite me attaching a full profile photo to my dating bio, men have still ended dates halfway through, citing my weight being the reason why they could no longer continue. I receive a flurry of fetishising messages from men who objectify my body and I have been the victim of the "Pull a Pig" prank, where a group of friends will pay a man money for daring to sleep with a fat woman.'

I remember reading an article that Yeboah wrote about her horrifying 'Pull a Pig' dating experience, where she was conned into going on a date with a man who had been dared to 'pull a fat chick' and was to receive a sum of money his friends had pooled if he completed the dare. It's beyond disgusting – I have no words that will do justice to just how horrendous that is and how that must have left Yeboah feeling. Reading her article, I was *stunned*, and it opened up my eyes to just a glimpse of what fat people face navigating this diet culture-ridden, fatphobic world: it is utterly dehumanising. I'm sad and ashamed that it took reading this for me to start to understand just how badly fat people are treated and how utterly draining and painful it must be. Luckily, Yeboah has done a lot of healing and work on her body image issues and is in a much better place today. She now shares beautiful lifestyle content alongside her self-love journey and is a fantastic Instagram follow, FYI.

While there are so many overtly cruel manifestations of fatphobia, sometimes, its presence can be more subtle, dressed up as 'concern' for the fat person: 'I'm just worried about your health' kind of comments and unsolicited weight-loss advice, aptly named 'concern trolling'.

Other examples of concern trolling include:

- 'I just want you to eat healthier'.

- 'I just think it's a good idea to watch your weight'.

- 'You're putting yourself at risk of medical conditions if you carry on like this'.

- 'Why don't you try taking up exercise?'

- 'You could try eating less junk'.

- 'I just care about you'.

This concerned attitude may originate from a place of believing that thinness equates to good health and fatness equates to bad health and so such comments can be well-

intentioned but their impact is overwhelmingly negative –
and counterproductive. Shaming people into losing weight
doesn't work: in a landmark study of 2,600 people, researcher
Janet Tomiyama discovered that being told 'you're too fat'
actually increased weight gain over time, as well as, of course,
disordered eating. Shame is not an effective motivator.

Other more subtle examples include refusing to sit next to a
fat person on the bus or congratulating a fat person on losing
weight and telling them that they look better for it (they don't,
they just look thinner). Or a thin person telling their fat friend
that they 'feel fat' (invariably in a way to convey that they
don't feel good about themselves because our collective fear
of fat makes that a deeply negative assessment).

So what's the solution? How can we combat this deeply ingrained
and insidious belief that fatness is something to be ashamed
of because it is the opposite of the beauty standard that we in
the West have had imposed on us for so long? 'Body positivity'
has been a huge topic of conversation over the past few years:
it is currently one of social media's biggest trending hashtags.
Sounds good, right? After a lifetime of diet culture, being positive
about our bodies has got to be a good thing. . . I absolutely
used to think so and, for a while, I proudly considered myself
to be part of the body positivity movement. I was changing
the conversation in my head about my body, overcoming
various eating disorders and very negative body image to get
to a better place – that sounded like body positivity to me.

But that's not what the body positivity movement is. Contrary to popular belief, saying 'I love my body' does not mean you are 'body positive' in the true sense of the term: don't get me wrong, it's fantastic and hopefully one day every person on this planet will be able to say 'I love my body', but it's more complicated than that. Body positivity has roots in fat acceptance, a radical political movement in the 1960s to liberate fat bodies. It was largely spearheaded by fat, Black women and women of colour as a safe space to exist in their own bodies, protected from a world where they were discriminated against and pushed to the margins of society.

With the rise of Instagram in 2012, women from all corners of the world were able to use the hashtag #bodypositivity to find other marginalised individuals, share support and advice and feel accepted. But as body positivity gained popularity, its meaning became distorted and people in socially acceptable bodies, like me, began to populate the hashtag.

This spiralled and, fast-forward to today, 'body positivity' has turned into a space dominated by privileged bodies and an advertising tool, commodified and adopted by brands for commercial gain using a very narrow vision of fatness: women with hourglass figures, flat stomachs and no cellulite that otherwise fit the standard of beauty apart from being a couple of sizes larger. The women are not marginalised, yet their images are used by companies to jump on the bandwagon of 'body positivity'. This leads to just another beauty ideal – one that is unattainable for most fat women, yet one that, they are told, now represents them in the media.

This shuts out fat people and especially larger fat people; those who are truly marginalised have been erased from the one place that they were safe in. Body positivity now centres on the experiences of people suffering from body image concerns, rather than the experiences of fat people, disabled people, Black people, people of colour and trans people fighting for the right to exist in a world inherently against them.

'Priority should be given to the bodies that have to deal with constant oppression and abuse on a daily basis, and that visibility should not be centred on bodies that benefit from societal body privilege,' says Stephanie Yeboah.

A lot of the people who the body positivity movement was made for no longer align themselves with body positivity – which is understandable. But it's important to recognise the origins of this now very mainstream movement and the ways in which it continues to ostracise people who needed it.

As someone who lives in a privileged body and publicly talks about body image, this is something that I have found particularly confronting. While I know I am helping a lot of women to feel better in their own skin, by encouraging body confidence and self-acceptance and denouncing beauty standards, I also know that there is no true body freedom until we are all free – and that includes dismantling fatphobia. For that reason, I make a concerted effort to educate my audience about fatphobia (using other people's experiences) and amplify the voices of marginalised bodies – but I am always willing to learn and contribute to making this world a little bit easier for fat people.

# So – for those of us who live in privileged bodies, what can we do? Here are some suggestions:

- Take a stand against fatphobia whenever you encounter it. No matter who it's against, no matter how subtle and even if you feel uncomfortable doing so, call it out. Report fatphobia on online platforms.

- Get comfortable with the word 'fat' and its use as a neutral descriptor.

- If someone refers to themselves as 'fat', don't try to correct them. Instead, work on ridding the negative associations of the word.

- Try not to call yourself fat if you are not.

- Avoid the words 'obesity' and 'overweight'.

- Seek out fat voices, like Aubrey Gordon, Roxane Gay, SJ Thompson and Sonya Renee Taylor, and listen to their experiences. Believe them and let them inform how you treat fat people.

- Ditch the diet talk. Anything that contributes to diet culture, that values thinness above all else, contributes to and perpetuates fatphobia. Also, it's damaging for fat people to hear constantly how hard people are trying to NOT look like them.

- Avoid commenting on people's bodies. Even if you think you're paying them a compliment, congratulating someone on losing weight reinforces the idea that fat = bad and thin = good.

- Avoid unsolicited health advice. Unless you're a doctor and they're your patient, someone else's health is none of your business.

- Remember that fat does not automatically mean unhealthy.

- Keep a check on your internal dialogue. Challenge yourself when an anti-fat thought comes up: question it and explore it before eliminating it.

- Advocate for more fashion choices for fat women with brands who refuse to cater for women above a certain size.

- Remember that fat people also suffer from eating disorders.

I really hope this chapter has shed some light on the critical importance of dismantling fatphobia, because it really is essential. Nobody deserves to be treated badly – or any differently to anyone else – for the way they look. And, as we discussed earlier, if fat people are to exist in a world without oppression, thin people need to shout loud and help make it happen.

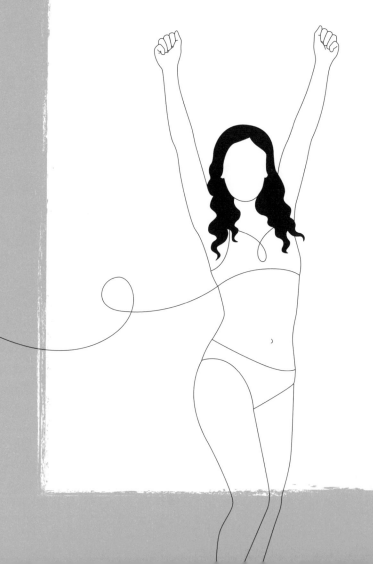

# CHAPTER 6

Beauty is only a trend

Who else remembers the book 'Does My Bum Look Big in This?'

As a teenager, I distinctly remember browsing at my local bookstore and spotting this title. It cemented little fragments of understanding I'd picked up from other places like TV, film, magazines and some adults in my life: it's not good to have a big bum; a pear shape is undesirable.

Back home, I stood with my back to the mirror and tried to turn my head as far as possible so I could see what my bum looked like – was it big? I wasn't really sure; it was something I hadn't previously considered. I ended up getting another mirror and angling it in front of me so I could get a full view of my rear end. I was lucky that this particular requirement didn't necessarily affect me, as someone with a distinctly average-sized derriere, but I imagine the realisation that BIG BUMS ARE BAD could have been very distressing for those with a shapelier behind.

Fast-forward 15 or so years and big bums have become the most celebrated body trend – with people the world over being encouraged to 'grow' their behinds, through exercise or otherwise. *TIME* magazine argues that this desire for curvier physiques has been at least partially driven by the global obsession with the Kardashians, as typified by the 2014 *Paper* magazine cover on which Kim poured champagne into a saucer balanced on her rear end. Many have compared this image of Kim to images of Saartjie Baartman, a nineteenth-century Black South African woman who was paraded in front of European audiences as an object of fascination, not celebration. Kim's leveraging (for her own gain) of aesthetic features that Black women have long been exoticised – and discriminated against – for having is not only an example of Blackfishing; it has also driven women, mainly young women, to stop at no lengths in trying to achieve a curvier physique (more on that soon).

What this demonstrates is that diet culture doesn't just capitalise on the notion that being 'thin' is the ultimate goal: every few years, a new 'ideal' body shape emerges and the goal posts shift. The new desirable shape is nearly always still thin but just with different characteristics (and more often than not Eurocentric characteristics, despite the multicultural world we live in) – and we're encouraged to covet this particular shape and achieve it no matter the risk, even if it is physiologically at odds with our own.

A couple of years ago, I took a picture of myself and photoshopped it according to the ideal body shape of each decade from the 1950s to today. The post went viral: it was shared thousands of times, I was contacted by multiple international news sources and I even appeared on a talk show in the US to discuss it. I was surprised at how quickly it spread but I think I know why: we're all either consciously or subconsciously aware that body trends exist and yet we usually let it go unquestioned. It's just the 'norm', something that is so deeply rooted in our culture that it isn't challenged. Seeing it laid out visually is confronting and really highlights the damage but I think it's also comforting – it is perfect proof that there is nothing wrong with our bodies; we just think there is because we're trying to make them conform to a warped perception of perfection that is ever-changing.

Body trends aren't a new phenomenon, they have existed for thousands of years. If we go back far enough and look at

There is nothing wrong with our bodies; we just think there is because we're trying to make them conform to a warped perception of perfection that is ever-changing.

sculptures from the Stone Age, we see that the desired body shape was fat, as supported by the artefacts like the famous Venus of Willendorf, a carving of a fat woman with big breasts. In Ancient Greece, Aphrodite, the goddess of sexual love and beauty, was often portrayed with curves.

As we explored in Chapter one, how a woman's body 'should' look has changed with practically each decade: from the hourglass shape of the Victorian era, widely achieved with the corset, to the 'heroin chic' thinness of the 1990s and back to hourglass – but this time more extreme – in 2010.

It was, however, the 1990s and early 2000s that had the most profound effect on my own body image. Young and without the wisdom, perspective or experience to understand that beauty trends and the ideal that is forced on us is going to change – just like fashion trends – I was heavily influenced by the glorification of 'size 0' and the 'heroin chic' aesthetic (very thin, accompanied by smudged eyeliner, messy, bedhead hair and pale skin). The 'size 0' craze (it was American and translates to a UK size 4, a 23-inch waist) had, no doubt, an impact on many – and the reason for its invention lies with vanity sizing. American designer Nicole Miller is unofficially credited with creating the size 0: 'One year, our sales manager wanted to size the clothes bigger and we started calling the size 8s a 6,' she told *The Hollywood Reporter*. 'Then the result of that was losing the smaller customer, so we had to add the zero. We also occasionally made some 00s.' Essentially, brands realised that the smaller the size that a shopper fits into, the more likely they are to buy, and they started to lower the numbers on their sizing. This created a need for size 0 and 00s and 'size 0' started to take shape as an ideal status symbol. It was perpetuated by ultra-thin celebrities including Nicole Richie, Lindsay Lohan and Mischa Barton and their stylist Rachel Zoe, who, very thin herself, was widely reported to refuse to work with any clients above a size 0. She vehemently denied these claims.

I don't think it's a coincidence that in 2011, anorexia nervosa was found to be the mental disorder with the highest rate of mortality.[24]

I idolised the bodies of certain models and celebrities: Kate Moss and the Olsen twins were my main sources of 'thinspiration' and I lived by Kate's (in)famous mantra: 'Nothing tastes as good as skinny feels.' I know, it pains me to write it. I just wanted to look like them and I resented the fact that my naturally curvy figure was so at odds with this 'ideal' that I wanted to achieve. I believe that this becoming so ingrained in me was a big part of the reason why I went on to have a breast reduction in my twenties, to attempt to look 'more straight up and down'. It's kind of hard to admit this (I made up excuses about severe back pain to those who questioned why I was having the procedure), but it's the truth. I don't regret the breast reduction – everything that I did makes up part of my story and the reason I do what I do today – but I do wonder if I would have been so compelled to undergo the procedure if curves had been celebrated when I was growing up and becoming aware of my body.

'Toned' was the buzzword in the early 2000s, with the rise in popularity of the Victoria's Secret show and their slender but sporty tanned figures, and Britney Spears sparked a craze for abs with her midriff-baring outfits. The incidence of eating disorders was reported to rise from 32.3 per 100,000 in 2000 to 37.2 in 2009 in the UK.[25]

Kim Kardashian and her family ushered in new curvy body ideals with their show *Keeping Up with the Kardashians*, which launched in 2007. By the 2010s, the body goal was an exaggerated hourglass figure – big breasts, a tiny waist, flat stomach and big hips. While many praised the Kardashians for showing women that they didn't have to be thin, they did, however, create a new and equally if not more unattainable ideal – and it's widely reported that they achieved their physiques using cosmetic procedures.

Kim has long been accused of sculpting her famous, internet-breaking derriere through the use of surgery, though she has vehemently denied all such allegations. Her denial hasn't stopped young girls and women from turning to such measures to emulate the star, though: the Brazilian bum lift (BBL) procedure, where liposuction is used to remove fat from the body (usually the stomach) before it goes through a purifying process outside of the body and reinjected into the hips and bum, was reported to have risen by 77.6 per cent from 2015 to 2020.[26]

In 2020 alone, there were 40,320 bum augmentations[27] – this includes both implants and fat grafting (BBL) – and according to Google keyword data, 'BBL' was searched around 200,000 times per month between January 2021 and May 2021.[28] These are shocking statistics – particularly when you consider the implications of the procedure. The healing process is long

and intense – patients are not allowed to lay on their backs
or sit directly on their bums for a minimum of three weeks
and are required to wear a skin-tight garment that reduces
swelling – but it's the death rate that's especially troubling. In
2018, the American Society of Plastic Surgeons estimated that
the BBL death rate was 1 in 3,000, making it 'a rate of death
far greater than any other cosmetic surgery'. This risk is down
to damage to blood vessels during surgery, which allows fat to
enter the bloodstream and causes a blockage of blood flow.

Standards had improved by 2020, when a study on the BBL
death rate estimating a rate of around 1 in 14,952.[29] Better, but
still a pretty horrifying risk, when you consider that the reason for
the surgery is purely aesthetic and in order to pursue a trend. This
is no judgement towards people who do decide on plastic surgery
– it's your body and it's your choice. I just believe that it's worth
unpacking your desire to have plastic surgery: does it come from
a place of self-loathing, from a deep-seated belief that your body
is wrong because you've been told so much and so often that it
is? It's worth exploring and unpicking to see if surgery is *really*
the answer (people often have surgery with the aim of improving
their self-esteem but find they aren't any happier afterwards).
But, it is your choice, so no judgement, and I mean that.

It is concerning that young women in particular are opting
for the BBL treatment in order to achieve a body trend that is
almost guaranteed to soon be out of fashion (maybe it already
is as you are reading this . . .). Because that's what happens
with all of these body trends, as history illustrates: they come
into fashion, they're coveted the world over and women go
to extreme lengths to achieve them, and then we move on to

something else. It's not fair on vulnerable, young women. I think of myself as a confused teen, suddenly terrified of having a big bum, then fast-forward only a decade or so and we are so convinced that we have to *have* big bums that people will risk life-threatening surgery for it. It goes to show just how spurious the whole pursuit of a trend is.

Social media has been instrumental in releasing the taboo of plastic surgery. With unprecedented access to our favourite celebrities and influencers, we are more cognisant of what goes on behind the scenes – including surgeries. This has removed the stigma and made it more ordinary and acceptable for non-celebrities to undergo procedures.

This is, unfortunately, heightened by the micro body trends that social media is responsible for creating and perpetuating to a worldwide audience. In the earlier years of Instagram, around 2013, the 'thigh gap' trend went viral and women looked to the space (or lack of space) between their thighs as a way to measure their 'beauty'.

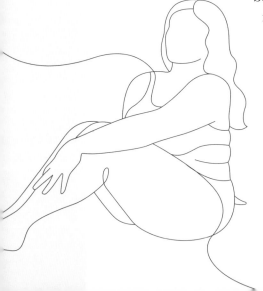

Shortly after, the 'bikini bridge' emerged, where bikini bottoms are suspended between the two hip bones, causing a space between the bikini and lower abdomen. I know, it sounds totally ridiculous, but it was a very real thing that spread across social media and prompted a flurry of 'bikini bridge' shots from celebrities and influencers – pictures that, previously, would have lived solely on pro-anorexia websites.

It was around this time that exercise fad The Skinny Bitch Collective (SBC) rose to social media prominence. Invented by personal trainer Russell Bateman, SBC was an invitation-only workout class championed by stars including Nicole Scherzinger, Ellie Goulding and Millie Mackintosh. Essentially, you had to be a celebrity or a model to take part and, while it was never explicitly stated that fat girls weren't allowed to join in, Russell was once quoted as saying: 'There's nothing interesting for me about making someone who's overweight a little bit less overweight.' There was certainly never any indication that anyone who wasn't 'skinny' had received an invite.

In a journalistic capacity, I once attended one of the classes. I was taken aback by the other girls in the session: tall, impossibly thin and toned – it felt like I was surrounded by Victoria's Secret angels. I left feeling pretty inadequate, even though I was at a fairly low weight myself at that point.

In 2015, there was a collective backlash against the 'skinny' ideal that had dominated social media and the focus shifted to 'strong': you know, the famous #strongnotskinny hashtag. Fitness influencers like Kayla Itsines shot to fame for her lean yet strong physique, with visible abs and muscly arms. She released an exercise regime, the Bikini Body Guide (BBG), to her millions of followers, including me, my colleagues and my friends, for a reasonably low price and without the requirement for special gym equipment so we could 'improve' our bodies at home. But the guide itself was convoluted and difficult to understand, and keeping on top of the routine was time-consuming. My friends and I had a WhatsApp group dedicated to our commitment to the programme. While I can't find any exact data on how many guides were purchased, it's reported that her platform sold for $430 million in 2021.

The #strongnotskinny or 'strong is the new skinny' phase was praised by many as a shift away from diet culture. But #strongnotskinny was simply diet culture dressed up in new clothes: rather than a focus on looking thin, there was an emphasis on looking thin *and* fit. Instead of a new diet telling you what and what not to eat, it was a personal trainer or a social media fitness influencer. Strength became another standard to conform to and a distraction from the fact that our culture is deeply fatphobic. This isn't surprising: diet culture is very clever at rebranding and #strongnotskinny is far from the only example – the 'wellness' trend is another. With diet advertising and marketing working tirelessly to keep up with the current trends and public opinion, it reinvents itself with the promise of empowering, all the while imposing more rules about what we're 'supposed' to look like.

Towards the end of 2015 and into 2016, fuller figures began to gain popularity. After Robyn Lawley was the first plus-size model to be featured in *Sports Illustrated*'s swimsuit issue and fashion designer Christian Siriano included five plus-size models in his show during New York Fashion Week, plus-size social media models like Iskra Lawrence, Ashley Graham and Hunter McGrady began to gain recognition. The hashstag #mermaidthighs began to trend, with users embracing their thicker thighs. While this was undoubtedly a positive move in many ways, most of these now-famous plus-size women had one thing in common: a fairly flat stomach, relatively slim arms and face and an hourglass physique. While it was liberating for many – including me – to see these women unapologetically embrace themselves, it continued to ostracise fat people who remained marginalised.

Because of course fat women are never 'in trend'. It's important to consider that while the 'plus-size' models like Ashley Graham became popular, their bodies are still socially acceptable. Fat people who suffer at the hands of a fatphobic society have never had their time in the spotlight: why? I suspect it's because we have been so conditioned to be anti-fat – so that diet culture, the belief that thinness is the best thing a human can achieve, and subsequently the diet industry, thrives, allowing people to continue profiting off our desire to be thin – that being fat is too far removed from what could be thought to be coveted. And so it never is.

Pro-anorexia content – also known as 'thinspiration' and usually online material that promotes thinness and behaviours related to anorexia – made a return in 2017, with the emergence of the visible ribcage as a trend, thought to be prompted by bikini photos of Bella Hadid with her ribs on display. Countless celebrities jumped on this trend, sharing their own take. The following year, the internet did itself proud with the emergence of a new thigh gap trend: the 'Toblerone tunnel'. I know, I can't believe I'm writing about this either, but here we are. Inspired by the famous triangular chocolate bar, the idea behind it is that people who possess a 'Toblerone tunnel' can fit a bar of Toblerone between their upper thighs. I . . . don't know what to

Diet culture is nothing
if not incredibly smart
at recognising a
'problem' and offering
a 'solution' – for a
price, of course.

say. While not endorsed by Emily Ratajkowski, the inspiration for this craze appeared to be the model's Instagram photos.

Thankfully, the 'Toblerone tunnel' phase didn't last long but 'slim thick' took over in 2019. According to the Urban Dictionary, this term describes 'a woman with big/toned thighs, plump booty, normal-sized hips and a flat/toned stomach'. Big thighs, but zero cellulite, of course. This look is embodied by Kim Kardashian, Beyoncé and J-Lo, and emulated by thousands of social media influencers, no doubt prompting the increase in plastic surgery rates as non-celebrities and non-influencers attempt to achieve the trending look. A microtrend originating from 'slim thick' was 'thigh brows' – thought to be sparked by Kylie Jenner, this is the curve that appears on top of the thighs as you sit. Again, I'm mostly speechless. And a bit confused.

As the Covid-19 pandemic struck the world in 2020, social media usage increased and video-sharing platform TikTok exploded in popularity, surpassing over 2 billion downloads worldwide as of April 2020. Less regulated than Instagram, which had certain filters in place to monitor triggering content, pro-anorexia content thrived on the app and teens started to take part in trends such as the A4 waist challenge, which deemed that your waist should not be visible beyond an A4 piece of paper while held up against it, and the collarbone challenge, which encouraged participants to see how many coins they could balance on their collarbones, the idea being that the more the collarbone sticks out, the more coins it's able to hold. Horrifying.

Most of these trends have been commodified: waist trainers surged in popularity after the 'slim thick' trend took over, promising to reshape your midsection using force (research has since emerged that the garments can damage vital organs and harm the digestive system but they're still incredibly popular – Selfridges even has a £74 version currently available to buy); fitness trainers sold guides specifically to attain a thigh gap and the diet industry sells thousands of products that promise to thin arms, get rid of cellulite and build abs. Because, you know, diet culture is nothing if not incredibly smart at recognising a 'problem' and offering a 'solution' – for a price, of course.

Researching and writing about these trends has been pretty depressing in many ways. Firstly, it starkly lays out just how much pressure we've had to contend with – think of the cumulative effect of internalising all these different ideals and beliefs about our body image.

Next up: where are these body trends for men? Yes, men are not immune from beauty standards and in recent years, they've been under pressure to become more ripped, undoubtedly leading to many problems with male mental health and self-esteem, but the focus on appearance is so unfairly skewed towards women. The patriarchy benefits from women being obsessed with how they look and every single new trend that emerges contributes to keeping us locked in a patriarchal society. This pursuit to attain a certain body ideal limits our capacity by taking up precious time, energy and money, meaning we're distracted from going out into the world and achieving what would actually be valuable and important.

Lastly, it's all just so . . . futile. All of it. Every single body trend we've explored on this page. Because what good does it serve?

How does meeting the trend of the moment enrich our lives? What value does it bring?! Especially when, in a certain amount of time, it will no longer be seen as desirable . . .

These trends all completely ignore the fact that we are all entirely unique and that is a *good* thing. We all have different DNA, different genes, and that is a wonderful part of humanity. Trying to manipulate our body according to what the celebrity *du jour* looks like strips away a part of our identity and attacks our sense of self. Not to mention leads to poor body image, self-esteem and potentially mental health issues.

We all look so wildly different and that's so incredible – imagine if we were all clones of each other, how utterly boring that would be? Diversity is beautiful and it should be celebrated in ALL of its different forms – all shapes and all sizes. We appreciate and value the diversity among flowers or, my preferred analogy, dogs (any Betty fans here?!). There are lots of different species of flowers and breeds of dogs and, while we might have one particular favourite, we see the beauty and joy in all of them. Why don't we see humans in this way? Because, I suspect, that if we did, we wouldn't have such a booming and lucrative diet industry and women would be more rebellious against the patriarchy.

The quest to construct a body that's close to what's in fashion takes us further away from what truly makes us happy. Diet culture and the patriarchy dictates that how we look is what defines happiness and success but this is not true. What really brings satisfaction is a meaningful life built on the connections we have with others. Once again, you're enough as you are, exactly as you are.

# CHAPTER 7

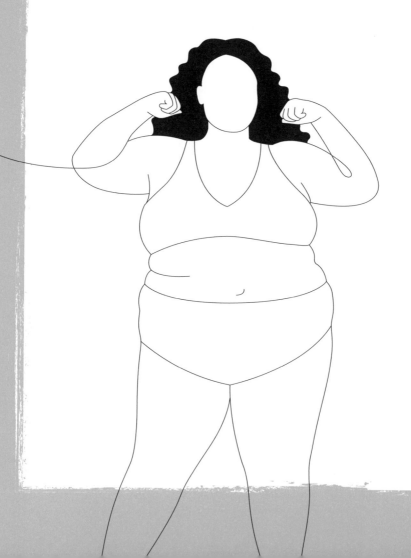

How you look
is the least
interesting
thing about you

# Are you happy with your body?

Or do you believe life will only truly begin when you 'fix' it – when you finally attain the 'perfect' body?

If that's how you feel, you're not alone: while it's very difficult to quantify a true percentage, studies suggests up to 91 per cent of women are dissatisfied with their body.[30]

As we've just discussed, ideal body trends change regularly, and often depend on which celebrity is currently most popular. But historically, trends have been centred around thin, cis-gendered, white, youthful and non-disabled, thanks to the extremely limiting, problematic and discriminatory standards of beauty that most of us have grown up around in the West. That's starting to change, but not fast enough.

So many of us have internalised those standards of beauty and the diet industry revolves around our desire to achieve them – no matter the means. The reward for achieving them, we've been taught, is happiness, success, desirability and lovability. Diet culture dictates that whatever the problem, losing weight and moving further towards the standard of beauty is the solution.

I used to believe that weight loss and happiness were synonymous, often reinforced by the euphoria I felt when I watched the numbers go down on the scale and reached a (arbitrary) goal I had set for myself. But this euphoria was only ever temporary, quickly replaced by a yearning for more, and this encouraged me to set and reach a new goal. I became trapped in this cycle, constantly wondering at which 'goal' I'd eventually feel content. Of course, I didn't, and I ended up in treatment for anorexia. I did what I thought I needed to do, what I'd been told I was supposed to do – reduce the size of my body – but it didn't make me happy, it made me sick and miserable. To the outside world, to those who didn't know me well, my life looked glamorous and happy and I probably looked happy with my body: I showed off my shrinking physique in tight clothes and wrote about fashion, and an outsider may well have believed I was living the 'dream' – which goes to show that you never know what's really going on with someone and thin really just does not equal happy. Mine is an extreme example, I know, but I think it illustrates how, when it's served to us by diet culture and damaging media practices with an agenda (making money), what we believe will make us happy rarely does.

However, at this point, I feel that it's important to acknowledge and confront something that feels deeply uncomfortable. While it's true that living in the kind of thin body we're taught to aspire to doesn't grant you immunity from life's struggles, it does mean that you're unlikely to experience appearance-based discrimination from others. Essentially, there is an argument that diet culture capitalises off knowing we get treated better when we're closer to whatever is currently deemed 'beautiful', so it works hard to heighten an individual's insecurities and offers a solution to ensure this happiness.

Happiness has long been linked to a particular body shape and size (thin) and weight loss in the Western world. Dr Sara Dowsett[31] is a chartered counselling psychologist and certified intuitive eating therapist specialising in body image dissatisfaction and disordered eating: 'The terms "weight loss" and "happiness" are often used synonymously by diet companies,' Dowsett points out. 'A quick scan of magazine front covers highlights this further: "Lose weight, get happy", "I lost 4st 13lbs and got my dream job" or "I'm a mum of two, I lost four stone and got my confidence back".' But, as she explains, the pursuit of lasting happiness is much more complicated than 'beauty' alone: 'If you keep manipulating your body through, for example, the process of restriction or cosmetic surgery to attain or sustain the "perfect" body, then yes, by default, you are automatically granted more privilege and acceptance from others and therefore a sense of happiness. But we need to question what the emotional, physical and financial cost to you is of a continual investment in the pursuit of beauty. Is it, for example, ever possible to reach a place where you can stop investing in your outward appearance or is this an ongoing pursuit that you must strictly adhere to in order to sustain your sense of happiness? And although you might be afforded certain privileges by meeting the "beauty ideal" and therefore avoid external discrimination from others, does it mean that you automatically avoid internal discrimination from yourself? Have you ever reached your target weight and received praise from others but still not felt content with your body? If you answered yes, that's because anytime we base our happiness on an external measure of worth, the reward will only ever be temporary.'

This is one of the most powerful statements around body image that I've ever read and it very succinctly summarises my experience: I was basing my happiness on something external and therefore seeking it in the wrong place. Happiness, I've come to believe, is not something that we can suddenly discover, but rather something to be uncovered within ourselves; something that is often squashed under layers of expectations, societal pressures and internalised, false beliefs. Does that make sense? I hope so. It does to me.

Happiness, I've come to believe, is not something that we can suddenly discover, but rather something to be uncovered within ourselves.

And at the risk of going too far off topic, I also think it's worth noting that happiness is not necessarily the state of euphoria we expect – and hope – it to be, but rather the absence of unhappiness. I found myself happier when I stopped thinking of happiness as euphoria or joy – of having incredible experiences and racking up achievements – and more like contentment: if there are no immediate concerns or stresses, I'm probably happy.

Being thin, or having the 'perfect body', was never going to bring me true, lasting contentment. This is backed up by social psychology, which highlights that beauty is not a strong predictor of lasting overall happiness or life satisfaction; it merely offers a temporary reprieve from diet culture-induced dissatisfaction with our bodies. Instead, research consistently reveals that the single biggest predictor of lasting human happiness is in the relationships and connections that we make in our life.[32]

Ironically, the pursuit of the 'perfect body' therefore must lead us further away from happiness. I know from personal experience that the time and energy we exert in trying to reshape our bodies is to the detriment of the relationships in our lives. The commitment is so all-consuming that we lack capacity to participate fully in our social lives; the dissatisfaction within ourselves drives us to be self-obsessed and reduces our amount of empathy for others.

I'd like to argue, also, that happiness is tied up with self-acceptance. If we now know that changing the way we look does not change how we *feel* about ourselves, surely the key is to accept ourselves as we are, warts and all. 'Happiness and self-acceptance go hand in hand,' according to psychologist Robert Holden, author of *Happiness Now!* 'The more self-acceptance you have, the more happiness you'll allow yourself to accept, receive and enjoy. In other words, you enjoy as much happiness as you believe you're worthy of.'

It is imperative that we believe we're worthy right now – and NOT when we've lost Xlbs and can fit into that dress. But this is difficult when we've been taught that we aren't unless we look a certain way.

'Working on repairing your relationship with your body after years of body image dissatisfaction is not a linear or quick process,' says Dowsett. She advises adopting a realistic approach: 'I find that clients tend to have a firm desire to love their bodies or to feel consistently confident, and while "love your body" is a much more positive message for children, young people and adults to hear, it is still problematic as it connects the body with a particular "goal". This goal poses a binary outcome – you either do love your body or you don't. But body image is a much more complex and multi-faceted issue that is in a constant state of ebb and flow, allowing for both good and bad body image days.'

Reframing a goal of 'body love' to a desire for 'body neutrality' or 'body respect' is a much more compassionate and realistic aim for people who have struggled with body image for their entire life. Body neutrality promotes accepting your body as it is and recognising its abilities and non-physical traits instead of its physical appearance: you may not love the way it looks or functions and that's fine, you don't have to, as long as this doesn't negatively impact your life and you appreciate the capabilities it does have. It encourages us to see our bodies in their most pure form: as a vessel to keep us alive and allow many of us to dance, swim, grow and birth children and feel joy. Its outward appearance plays no part in how it functions. Body neutrality promotes taking a neutral view of your body without any requirements of self-love talk or mantras about your body. Personally, I found huge relief in the body neutrality movement. Attempting to 'love' my body was proving difficult after spending such a long time at war with my appearance, but neutrality seemed much more attainable. I saw it as making peace with my body and it gave me a renewed sense of determination, as well as an understanding that the body's primary function is to keep us alive and allow us to navigate life, not to look a certain way.

*So body neutrality is our goal.*

And if you are able to progress to self-love and fall in love with how your body looks – great! If not, that's OK too. So how do we go about reaching body neutrality? 'It must start with a deliberate and conscious intent to break free from diet culture and it is essential that you receive appropriate support along the way to do so,' says Dowsett.

If we're wrapped up in diet culture, we'll never make peace with our bodies – something I learnt first-hand from multiple failed attempts. I wanted to heal the relationship with my body while still believing I needed to lose weight in order to do so. But despite my conviction that dieting and body acceptance was not mutually exclusive, I found that the first time I started making *real* progress with how I perceived my body was when I finally put weight on the backburner.

So, how to do this? 'Whenever I begin working therapeutically with clients to repair their relationship with their bodies, I always find it necessary to start with the unlearning of their old, unique beliefs and conditioning rather than immediately applying new learning to these old wounds,' says Dowsett. 'Exploring and acknowledging an individual's own narratives, scripts, personal stories and experiences associated with their body image dissatisfaction is an essential part of this therapeutic work.'

This might start with prompting questions such as: 'When did you first become aware of disliking your body?' or 'Can you recall earlier negative experiences at home or school where you felt your body was judged by others?' Many of the beliefs that shape how we feel about our bodies are formed during childhood, absorbed from people around us and adopted from

Many of the
beliefs that
shape how
we feel about
our bodies are
formed during
childhood.

the culture we grew up in; these questions often provoke an emotional response in us and bring to the surface any past personal experiences that have contributed to poor body image.

As part of these explorations, Dowsett is also keen to understand an individual's relationships with their primary caregivers – typically parents or grandparents – and how such relationships have contributed to their sense of self and body image. 'If I am working with an individual who identifies as female, then I will be curious to know, for example, what her mother's relationship with her own body and food is like and was like growing up. What template did she set for her daughter? Did the individual witness her mother on and off diets during childhood? Maybe the mother skipped meals in the pursuit of weight loss or rationed food because money was tight. Did she hear her mother talk positively or negatively about her body? Did her mother get into the water with her daughter on family holidays or did she stay stood on the sideline because of her own fear of her body being judged?'

The point of this exercise is not to attribute blame to parents – it's crucial to understand that they themselves have been subject to their own conditioning caused by the personal and societal messaging that they received in their upbringing. Rather, these explorations can help to pinpoint key contributors to body image dissatisfaction. 'It is only from a place of clarity with any mental health issues that the unlearning and healing can begin,' says Dowsett.

Once the personal origins of body image dissatisfaction are brought to the surface, the second step in the therapeutic process is for the individual to understand how these are part of a much larger oppressive societal system of power. 'It is impossible to talk about your dislike of your outward appearance without talking about wider systemic, oppressive issues at play,' says Dowsett. 'Issues such as racism, sexism, capitalism, classism, fatphobia or homophobia continue to inform and perpetuate your own personal perspective of your body within our society.' If you aren't compliant with the society 'standard', you may face discrimination and be marginalised. This threat creates a fear of looking outside of the 'norm' and so we subconsciously strive to be as obedient as possible – which explains why we are so fearful of getting fat.

Cognitive behavioural therapy (CBT) is a talking therapy often used in the therapeutic process to highlight the role that all of these negative cognitions play in maintaining body image dissatisfaction so we can subsequently unpack them and employ new behaviours. Therapy is a privilege that not many people are able to access but, luckily, self-directed CBT can be very effective. If you are unable to afford therapy to assist you in repairing your relationship with your body, Dowsett advises carrying out behavioural experiments like the following example with the help of affordable online resources (such as her 'Debunking Diet Culture' online course available at www.intuitivepsychology academy.com).

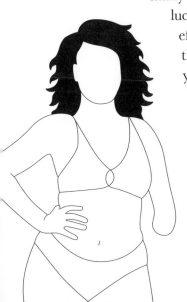

Dowsett explains that when a negative experience arises that is connected to our body image, four interconnected aspects of the self are activated: our physiological reactions (bodily sensations), our thoughts, our emotions and our behaviours.

Let's now refer to the behavioural experiment to illustrate this in action using a triggering experience that I imagine many of us have experienced at some point in our lives: a trip to the beach on a hot day. You might not go in the first place, through fear of how your body looks. If you do go, you arrive at the beach, it's warm and your friends start getting changed into their bikinis. What do you imagine is going on emotionally for you? Potentially you're experiencing worry, frustration or sadness. These emotional reactions have a physical impact on you: maybe a raised heart rate, a clenched jaw, a tightness in your chest or sweaty palms. Simultaneously, there will be a series of automatic thoughts that are racing, such as: 'I can't take this dress off and show my body', 'Everyone will be looking at my body' or 'I can't let them see me with my bikini on'.

The interplay between your bodily reactions, emotional reactions and thoughts results in a set of behaviours that will be automatically implemented as a way to manage and protect yourself from the discomfort – i.e. staying covered up, avoiding group photos or putting a stop to your trip altogether. 'While these may temporarily relieve the negative feelings, the persistent use of these "safety behaviours" actually perpetuates and maintains the vicious cycle of body image dissatisfaction. So it's these behaviours that need to be gently challenged in order to interrupt the cycle and provide you with alternative templates of experience,' says Dowsett.

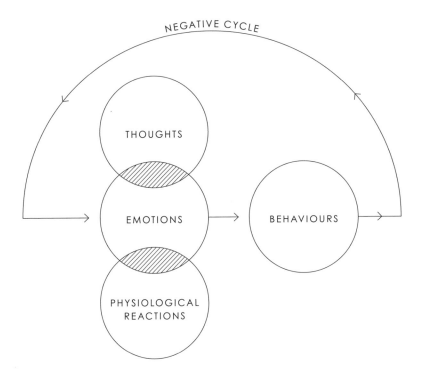

NEGATIVE CYCLE

THOUGHTS

EMOTIONS → BEHAVIOURS →

PHYSIOLOGICAL
REACTIONS

Essentially, we are to challenge ourselves and interrupt our behavioural patterns using gradual exposure and taking it step by step. This can, ultimately, help you to alter your automatic negative thoughts, emotions and bodily reactions.

In this particular scenario, this may look like simply deciding to go to the beach. You may feel your anxiety peak for the first 30 minutes but then it starts to reduce and you even find that there are some chunks of time where you aren't even thinking about your body. You realise nobody is actually looking at your body and you *might* even go into the sea for the first time in years! Perhaps you're not confident enough yet to get in the photos with your friends but you are proud of yourself for making this big first step.

As well as gaining a sense of confidence and pride from achieving something you thought wasn't possible, carrying out these CBT behavioural experiments challenges thoughts and beliefs, such as your friends judging your body, and increases your window of tolerance. It is a powerful method in bringing about change and leads to neuroplasticity. Neuroplasticity is the brain's ability to change itself by creating new neural pathways and alter existing ones, and it requires practice and repetition, so the more you challenge your current negative thoughts and behaviours around your body image, the quicker you will be able to replace them with positive ones.

In summary, Dowsett recommends adopting a multi-layered approach to this deep-rooted and complex issue. It begins with understanding your personal relationship with your body, along with any life experiences that may have informed it, followed by an unlearning of how you've been conditioned by wider systems outside of yourself to dislike and disown your body and finishing with challenging your thoughts, mindset and behaviour to bring about concrete changes that result in *lasting* change.

*A lot to take in, right?*

I know. And it doesn't need to be all at once. This process was a really slow burn for me – when I first started to explore the beliefs I held around my body, I was stunned to find just how many there were and just how deep they ran: I had once been called 'moonface' and it had cemented a complex about the size of my face; I had been told that I had 'legs like the footballers on TV' (I wish we could print a laughing emoji because that's what I'd like to add right now – what a bizarre thing to say to a kid?!) because they were muscly and, most painfully, that I was never going to be 'thin enough'. Writing them out now I feel almost trivialises them – having a big face doesn't sound like the end of the world, right? Neither does having muscly legs . . . but these beliefs really hampered my self-esteem. Which makes perfect sense: young girls are taught that the most important thing about them is how they look. Then they're told that how they look is inadequate, that it doesn't quite 'match up' – that's going to sting, isn't it?

The beliefs were all painful to uncover, and I wasn't able to access them all at once – many were so ingrained in me that I didn't even know they weren't real. I had never even so much as thought to question them.

And I was lucky enough to have access to therapy. So, please, be patient with yourself; for many of us, there is a lifetime of negative thought patterns to unpick and unlearn.

*But there's no better time to start than now.*

# CHAPTER 8

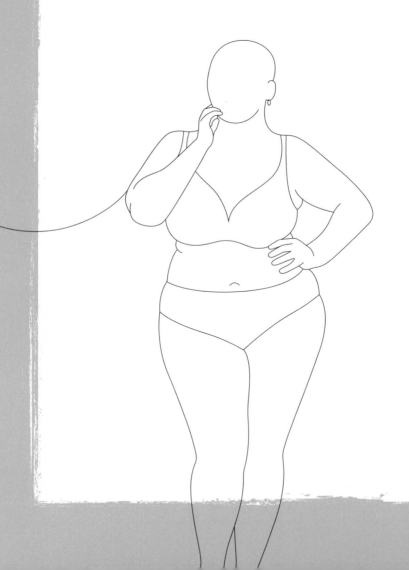

Comparison always leads to self-criticism

# 'Why don't I look like her?'

I think all of us have, at some point, wished we looked like someone else – whether it's a friend, a colleague, a model or a celebrity.

Body comparison can often be very debilitating, especially for people with body image dissatisfaction, which is why I've decided it's worthy of an entire chapter in this book. It is something I have struggled with my entire life: I have compared my body to almost every single woman I've ever seen – in real life, in magazines, on screen or on social media.

When I was at university, my friend introduced me to a website that listed the weights of practically every person who is and ever has been in the public eye. I knew, deep down, that it wasn't going to be helpful (or truthful – where did this information come from?) but I was still hooked: my own weight firmly at the forefront of my mind, I would spend hours poring over the website looking for celebrities who weighed the same as or less than me. The compulsion to do this was multi-faceted: my body dysmorphia meant that I had genuinely no idea how I looked and I was desperately trying to seek clarity through comparison; I was searching for reassurance that my current size was acceptable (I thought that if celebrities weighed a similar amount as me, that would mean it was OK) and I was using people with lower weights than me as 'motivation'. Looking back, I feel so sad for that young girl, so lacking in self-validation that I was desperately seeking approval through weight comparisons with celebrities.

I know I wasn't alone in this; I speak to so many people who feel trapped in body comparison and wracked with feelings of crushing inadequacy.

This wouldn't be so prevalent if a standard of beauty didn't exist. Imagine a world where we weren't taught that how we look is our most important asset and how we look had to be thin . . . A world where no body shape or size was valued over any other, where all appearance was just neutral: the concept of measuring up just wouldn't be relevant as there would be nothing to 'measure up' to.

But we don't. We live in a world where, as we know, the standard of beauty is deeply ingrained in the fabric of our culture and, therefore, is a collective priority. This is compounded by the fact that comparison is very much a hard-wired human tendency and evolutionary trait. As social animals, in our past, fitting in with the collective was important to an individual's survival. 'Comparison used to serve us well as a way to judge how safe we were, so we could make good decisions and survive: for example, as we developed into human civilisations, comparing our tracking skills to another member of the hunt could help us assess where we might need to hone our skills to stay as a valued member of our collective,' says Lucy Sheridan, the Comparison Coach.

So while it was initially helpful, Sheridan explains that comparing ourselves to others has turned into more of a compulsion, due to a variety of factors that are now inherent in our habits and society. 'From the very moment you are born, your size and weight are logged and charted against other babies. Then, as you progress through younger years, learning and development milestones are tracked against others'.' The feedback loop of our parents, teachers, caregivers and other adults of influence then starts to play a part and it cements our tendency to evaluate ourselves against those around us. Then, as we learn the importance of our appearance in society, we become aware of advertising featuring airbrushed models and celebrities with unattainable bodies that are widely considered 'beautiful'. We also hear our parents or trusted adults talk about their own bodies disparagingly and scrutinise the ways in which it doesn't match up to what it 'should', and another comparison is born.

Social media heightens this phenomenon. Ubiquitous, loud and chock full of everyone's best sides, it is a veritable breeding ground for comparison, offering up frequent and ample opportunity to feel that we are lacking. We lose sight of the fact that we are consuming a deliberately curated, filtered and edited one-dimensional view of someone's entire life, which is dangerous.

It's also particularly dangerous for people with low self-esteem or who have a negative body image because social media, with its visual nature, offers endless opportunity for women to seek out images depicting the thin ideal that used only to be available via traditional advertising. I don't think it's a coincidence that my use of Instagram skyrocketed as my eating disorder began to take a firm grip on me.

Back in the 1950s, psychologist Leon Festinger coined the term social comparison theory, which was the idea that people evaluate their own abilities and attitudes in relation to those of others. Essentially, that in order to gauge our own success, intelligence and appearance, we look to other people as points of reference. Three types of social comparison are proposed in the theory that I will refer back to:

1. **Upward social comparison**, which is comparing ourselves to those we perceive to be better than us.

2. **Downward social comparison**, which is comparing ourselves to those we perceive to be worse off than us.

3. **Lateral social comparison**, which is comparing ourselves with another who we consider to be more or less equal.

There is discussion around the advantages of comparison, with many believing that upward comparison can lead us to feel inspired and motivated. I'm not an expert but this doesn't sit right with me, from my own personal experience. Comparison is a game in which there is no endpoint because there is *always* someone who has more than you. And, I believe, it ties your happiness to a goal that is often very arbitrary: it doesn't really *mean* anything. You know how it goes: 'I'll be happy if I start earning this much money' or 'I'll be happy when I get this promotion'. Yes, these are positive things, but endlessly striving for them means that you are forever looking forward and failing to acknowledge and appreciate what you have, that you can be already happy with exactly what you have right now. And – I'm sure you'll have experienced this too – there is a very real danger that you achieve the goal and, rather than feeling the rush of happiness you spent so long working towards earning, you find yourself focusing on a new goal. The cycle then continues.

By turning outward, we also end up focusing on everyone else but ourselves – and what is right for someone else is not necessarily right for us. We might find ourselves setting off in pursuit of things that, we might realise with time to focus on ourselves, aren't really what we want.

There is also discussion around the advantages of downward comparison – the theory that comparing what you have to someone who has less than you can make you feel better about yourself. First off, this requires that we take pleasure in someone else's perceived misfortunes in order to buoy ourselves, and this mentality values competition over connection. You are devaluing others in order to value yourself.

Moreover, this once again places your validation and your contentment in the hands of someone else. What happens when that person goes on to get more than you? Then you'll feel worse about yourself. I experienced this first-hand several times when I compared myself to people who were bigger than me. I found temporary relief in the fact that I was thinner than some people. It pains me to admit that I used to do this – mainly because it was totally based in fatphobia and it was cruel – but I recognise that this is a common symptom of diet culture: we are constantly encouraged to compare when a standard of beauty is promoted to us and the media amplifies this. So, if you do this, too, you're not a bad person: it's just conditioning and we can undo that.

A few of the people I used for downward comparison ended up losing weight and becoming thinner than me. That immediately destabilised me and shook my sense of self.

Which I now realise doesn't make sense *at all* – what could someone else's weight possibly have to do with me, let alone my value as a person?

Comparison is something that I've worked on extensively because I don't want my sense of self to be built on something external. American inspirational speaker Iyanla Vanzant sums it up perfectly: 'Comparison is an act of violence against the self.' I believe that it takes away our power, fosters judgement and jealousy and can lead to ugly behaviour, like purposefully putting down others whom you consider superior to you as a way to boost your own self-esteem. I don't condone this behaviour, of course, but it's easy to see how we end up in such a dark place – diet culture and the patriarchy fuel this, especially for women, and it's vital that we don't blame ourselves for it and let it induce shame. Comparison can damage relationships, if we allow it to create distance between us and the people who make us feel inadequate. That person does not deserve to bear the brunt of our frustrations: our insecurities born of comparison are about us, not about them, and the only way they can be resolved is through internal work. So it's imperative to be conscious of them and to identify where the comparisons stem from.

Don't get me wrong – I am human and comparison will always be there for me, but I don't fight that; I strive instead to recognise it and work on it wherever I can (we'll explore how in a minute).

While the upsides of comparison are up for debate, the disadvantages are abundant and backed up by science: research has found that comparing fuels feelings of envy, low self-confidence and even depression.[33] 'For some, it might be that comparisons cause a bit of irritation and envy, which can be brushed under the carpet but still mount up insidiously over time,' says Sheridan. 'On the other end of the scale, comparisons can lead to a downward spiral of self-criticism that can keep someone gripped in a state of doubt and low confidence.'

This can be incredibly toxic for our relationships in lots of different areas – like career and romance – and I've spoken to many of you who admit to wanting to stay away from friends or family members who might be thinner than you because they make you feel inferior. It's dark territory and it can take over your life.

While comparison with others is toxic and requires healing, we can't forget the comparisons we make with ourselves.

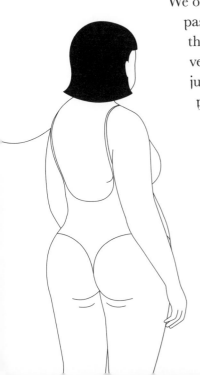

We often compare ourselves to our past selves – 'Why can't I still be thin like that?' – and an idealised version of ourselves – 'Why can't I just be *better*?' This is a sinister and paralysing comparison that feels particularly frustrating because we have evidence that something is possible for us because we had it previously. It feels more tangible.

I spent years grieving my previous, thinner body. I couldn't understand why I wasn't able to recreate my previous 'self-control' and 'motivation'. The problem? My previous body wasn't down to self-control or motivation; it was a result of an eating disorder and a lifetime of disordered eating. Yet I wasn't able to register that, I was simply blinded by frustration that I knew it was possible but I couldn't 'achieve' that again.

I think we all do this in one way or another when we idolise a past version of ourselves: we forget the surrounding circumstances. Ironically, often our past selves that we hold up against how we are now weren't particularly happy people enjoying a great time. It's worth exploring that when doubt next creeps in – don't look back with rose-tinted glasses.

A great way to combat comparison with ourselves is to reframe the negative thought; my therapist at the time, when I was struggling, taught me this. For example, she encouraged me to consider that yes, I was thinner, but I was also lacking in energy and concentration, both of which impacted my work and life as a whole; I was unable to enjoy a social life and I was deeply unhappy. This is an extreme example, I know, but I promise there is power in finding even the slightest glimmer of positivity: if you have gained weight by ditching dieting – well, you've given yourself food freedom, and that's *incredible*. Find your silver lining, hang on to it and allow it to soothe you when things feel hard.

*Enough talk about comparison, let's explore how we can avoid it.*

I spent years grieving my previous, thinner body.

The first thing I'd love for you to know is that comparison really is futile. Hopefully I've gone some way towards convincing you of this, if you didn't already agree. I am me and you are you, and there will never be another one of either of us – no two people in the world are identical and look identical. And there are many, many different reasons for this, including the fact that we all have different DNA, environments, upbringings, mental health, physical health and cultures. We are so, so incredibly unique and that is a special thing.

When you consider that we are all genetically predetermined to look completely different, it becomes even clearer just how unfair it is that we are encouraged to compare our body to someone else's, doesn't it? When I was younger and spending precious time and energy sizing up my weight against hundreds of different celebrities, it wasn't a true comparison. And when you compare your body to another, it's also not a true comparison. Why would you compare a rose to a tulip? They're both beautiful but they're not really comparable apart from the fact that they're both flowers!

*Remember that you, exactly as you are, are enough. And you are so much more than your body.*

I say this a lot and it's absolutely true, but I know it's difficult to fully believe when comparison strikes. And it's not always an easy thing to tackle – after years of programming thanks to diet culture and the patriarchy, it can be a process and each of us has our own complexities that require some self-analysis – but there are some actionable tips to help stop comparison in its tracks:

- **Sit with the comparison.** When you notice yourself having these thoughts, rather than attempt to bat them away, observe and acknowledge them. Then try going deeper to explore why this might have come up; usually, the comparison points to something we feel we're lacking in our own lives and it's powerful to get to the bottom of that. Once you understand it, you can take action. For example, 'I want to be as thin as her' likely indicates that you have some work to do with your body image.

- **Step back and broaden your lens.** Essentially, try to find perspective. 'It's so easy to fixate on one part of our body or physical feature and yet you are an incredible miracle,' says Sheridan. 'Start to shift your focus to looking at your broader life with some love and attention and set intentions and goals that inspire you to really connect with your life on a deeper level. This will help you see and build your feelings of how enough you feel are, which will start to create a shift in you and allow you to have more self-compassion and grace.'

• **Practise gratitude.** Gratitude journaling has long been advised as an effective way to avoid comparison. Taking a few moments to write down the things that you feel grateful for helps to shift your mindset from a place of comparison to a place of appreciation. I didn't do this for the longest time – I thought it was a bit too 'woo woo' for me – but I was sent a gratitude journal, decided to give it a go and the positive impact was almost instant.

• **Curate your online space**. As I said, social media is a breeding ground for comparison and if there are people who routinely prompt you to make a comparison with yourself, it's time to cull. It's vital that our feeds are a safe space. (We're going to explore this in depth in Chapter 12.)

• **Talk about it.** Sharing our struggles and being vulnerable with someone we trust can be very powerful – it provides support, deeper understanding and a sense of connection.

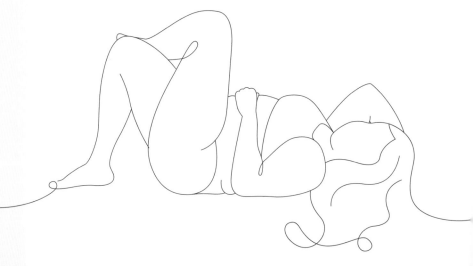

- **Mind how you speak to yourself.** We are our own worst critics and examining our self-talk can often be illuminating – what do you tell yourself that you would never say to someone you care about? What is the narrative in your head when you're making a comparison?

- **Take a break from people who do not support your growth.** 'There are some people in our lives who add to and reinforce our insecurities and the toxic habits that keep us comparing ourselves,' says Sheridan. 'We need to take responsibility for the role they play in our lives and make adjustments: if there are some WhatsApp groups where the conversations are all around physical fixations then perhaps mute them for a while; if certain work colleagues only talk about macros and calorie-counting, start seeing a bit less of them socially. Clean up your energy, take back your focus and your time so you can invest it back in yourself.'

There will always be people who have what you perceive to be a better body than yours, or who seem to be achieving things you wish you could, but the key is identifying what you have and the unique value that you bring to the world.

*All I can do is say it once more: you are enough. Exactly as you are.*

# CHAPTER 9

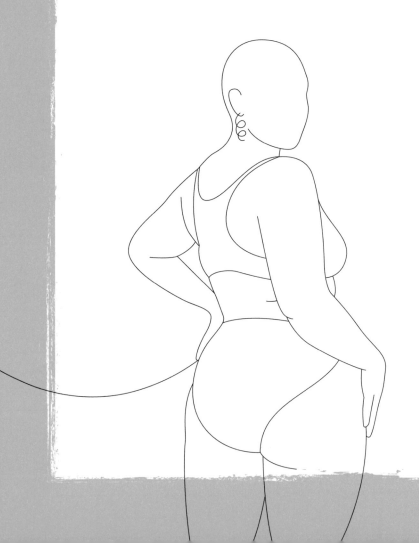

How we
*should*
be eating

# Has dieting dominated a huge part of your life?

If you're reading this book, I imagine the answer is 'yes'.
I think we've sufficiently covered why dieting is bad but here's
a brief reminder to take us into this more practical section:

- The vast majority of diets don't work; studies have shown
  that it is near impossible to keep off any weight initially lost.

- Diets affect your relationship with food and lead to
  disordered eating . . .

- They can also lead to full-blown eating disorders.

- Dieting slows down metabolism.

- Fad diets in particular often encourage you to consume
  very few calories, which can lead to physical problems.

- Anything that forces you to ignore your body's natural
  hunger cues is not a healthy and sustainable option.

So we need to ditch dieting – agreed? Great. But after a lifetime
of trying to follow the latest food-plan trend and/or sticking to
food rules that have been picked up from various different fad
diets, where on earth do we start?

I found this incredibly hard. I cannot emphasise enough just
how difficult this process was for me. During my recovery, I
was offered help from a dietitian at many points but I always
refused it because I truly believed I knew what I should be

eating. I thought that because I knew I should be eating only complex carbs and lots of vegetables, I was doing fine. It wasn't until much later down the line, when my therapist insisted I would receive great benefit from getting nutritional advice and I booked in an initial session with a dietitian, that I realised just how warped my relationship with food was.

I believed, for example, that carbs were only meant to be consumed with one meal per day. It sounds crazy writing this now but I genuinely believed it – it was a rule that I had picked up and internalised through doing every single low-carb diet I had ever managed to get my hands on. I also believed that you only needed two meals per day and that you should save eating things like chocolate, sweets and crisps until weekends – there should be a weekly 'cheat day' where you were allowed to eat the things that had been banned during the week. I had got this, no doubt, from various bits of 'advice' I had read online or seen in magazines or on TV.

Essentially, I had to start again, from scratch, and I was utterly confused. My dietitian, Aleeza Rosenberg, was kind and patient and not surprised: she had seen this many times before as a result of years of ingrained diet culture. We started with learning about food and different food groups – why you need them, how often to eat them and roughly how much of them to eat. Aleeza showed me a sample plate which gives a general guideline as to what you should be eating. And yes, carbs were included with each meal. My mind was blown and I was scared – I was scared that if I started to eat as she was suggesting, it would result in weight gain. Because carbs = weight gain, right?

Nope. Carbs are not the devil and they are not the root cause of weight gain. Crazy, I know. We have diet culture to blame for that belief.

I'm not going to say what happened with my body as far as weight fluctuation goes when I started eating as Aleeza was suggesting because I don't think it's helpful. If I say I lost weight, it will, consciously or subconsciously, translate to you as a diet just dressed up in different clothing. And if I say I gained weight, it will be a reason for you to fear ditching the diet. The truth is that either can happen – but we'll get on to that.

It's also somewhat beside the point, because the most important thing that resulted from my dietitian sessions was a much-improved relationship with food. I managed to dump the rules that had been skewing how I ate and focus on actually nourishing my body. Moving from thinking about food in terms of how to control my weight to using food to nourish my body and make me feel good was a very powerful mindset shift. Because food is so much more than whether it makes us thinner, fatter or maintains our weight – but at the same time, for most of us, the saying 'food is fuel' is very reductive. Food is enjoyment, self-care, tradition, culture, privilege and social connection.

Eating breakfast, lunch AND dinner, along with snacks as needed to level out my blood sugar in between, was so foreign to me, but so wonderful. It gradually alleviated a sense of doom that had clouded me for a long time, along with a constant feeling of fatigue. It made me feel stronger and it allowed me to focus and think more clearly.

I need to reiterate: it wasn't an overnight process. Even when I thought I was approaching meals in a healthy, balanced way, I was still actually restricting without knowing it – which at times lead to binge-eating or a loss of control around food. Aleeza had to point this out several times and I was genuinely surprised: I hadn't imagined that attempting to eliminate diet culture from my life would be *so* hard. I also had very little concept of my hunger and fullness: I had purposefully ignored these cues since I could remember and so they were totally out of practice. It took a long period of mindful eating to understand the signals that my body was trying to convey to me.

I must also stress that my eating isn't perfect now – and I think it might always be a work in process, something that I will always have to think about and keep in the back of my mind. I might be wrong, and it will be lovely if I am, but I've made peace with that: my background is so heavily dominated by eating disorders and disordered eating that I think it might be something that I continue to carry around to some degree. And that's OK; I am so happy with the progress that I've made and the fact that my life is not dominated by what I can and can't eat, and a constant obsession with food.

Why am I telling you this? It's not to discourage you – quite the opposite. I've seen some people say online that they ditched the diet, found peace with food and that their relationship with food is now basically perfect. Easy. But that didn't actually help me at all: reading that just set a standard that felt unachievable for me and made me feel like a failure when I couldn't meet it, which discouraged me from continuing. I know now that my brain works better focusing on a more realistic, day-by-day approach. It's also vital to acknowledge that food is a privilege for many who lack financial resources – having access to it may be difficult for some.

The point I want to make is that diet culture is very real and very overbearing and we live in a diet culture-dominated world, so wherever you end up is OK – whether you completely heal your relationship with food and never have to even think about it ever again, or whether you get to a better, healthier place with food but still have to pay attention to it.

So, with that in mind, enough about me, let's get on to you.

## How can you ditch the diet for good and work on healing your relationship with food?

I called on Aleeza herself for expert advice. First off, let's get to grips with what a healthy relationship with food looks like, which I believe can be illustrated using the principles of intuitive eating. Intuitive eating is a way of choosing what to eat that promotes a healthy, non-diet culture-based attitude towards food and body image. The movement was kickstarted by dietitians Evelyn Tribole and Elyse Resch, who, in 1995, published a bestselling book with the same name that has served a bible for people all over the world wanting to improve their relationship with food.

Here are the ten principles Evelyn and Elyse set out:

## 1. REJECT THE DIET MENTALITY

The diet mentality is the idea that there's a diet out there that will work for you and help you lose weight once and for all – which, as we now know, is very unlikely, so it's imperative that diets are banished. Intuitive eating is an anti-diet: nothing is off-limits and nothing is prescribed; you are simply encouraged to explore how your own relationship with food works best.

## 2. HONOUR YOUR HUNGER

Hunger is not your enemy. Respond to your early signs of hunger by feeding your body and keeping it biologically fed with adequate energy. If you let yourself get excessively hungry, this will probably trigger a primal drive to eat and you are likely to eat past fullness.

## 3. MAKE PEACE WITH FOOD

Quit the war against food; food is not your enemy. Give yourself permission to eat and challenge ideas about what you 'should' or 'shouldn't' eat.

## 4. CHALLENGE THE FOOD POLICE

Food is not good or bad – it is just food – and you are not good or bad for what you eat or don't eat. Food is not a moral issue; challenge thoughts that tell you otherwise.

## 5. RESPECT YOUR FULLNESS

Just as your body sends signals that it is hungry, it also tells you when it's full. Be attentive to the signals of comfortable fullness – which may well be subtle at the start of your journey – and, as you're eating, check in with yourself to see how the food tastes and how hungry or sated you're feeling.

## 6. DISCOVER THE SATISFACTION FACTOR

Remember that food is pleasure! This can get lost when we focus solely on how it makes us look but it is an experience that it supposed to be enjoyed, so make your eating experience enjoyable. Sit down to eat a meal that tastes good to you and enjoy it.

## 7. HONOUR YOUR FEELINGS WITHOUT USING FOOD

This is a difficult one. Evelyn and Elyse use this pillar to explain that emotional hunger will only mask the underlying issue and, ultimately, make you feel worse, so you should look to other ways of coping with your feelings. While this is often the case, especially for people who suffer with binge eating disorder, I believe it to be more nuanced, and the demonisation of emotional eating is perhaps not entirely helpful. Emotional eating can be a perfectly acceptable tool to cope with intense or uncomfortable emotions *if* you are making an intentional decision: you might have had a really rough week at work and you want to chill on the sofa with your partner and a big pizza; if you're feeling disconnected from someone special in your life, bonding over a hearty meal might feel really good; and if you've got your period and you're feeling emotional and hormonal, a bar of chocolate is sometimes the best cure. But when food is your *only* coping mechanism, eating to soothe isn't an intentional decision: it's simply the only tool in your arsenal and in that case, it would likely be helpful to call on other ways of coping. Evelyn and Elyse suggest finding ways that are unrelated to food to deal with your feelings, such as taking a walk, meditating, journaling or calling a friend. It might also be helpful to identify when a feeling that you might call hunger is actually based on emotion.

## 8. RESPECT YOUR BODY

Accept your genes. You wouldn't expect someone with a shoe size of six to squeeze into a size four, right? So let's get rid of those expectations about our bodies. We are who we are and there's beauty in that. Rather than judging your body for how it looks and what you perceive is wrong with it, recognise it as capable and beautiful just as it is.

## 9. EXERCISE – FEEL THE DIFFERENCE
Forget everything you've been fed by the diet and fitness industries and find ways to move your body that you enjoy (we'll explore this in more detail in Chapter 12). Shift the focus from losing weight and manipulating your body with exercise to using it to feel energised, strong and alive.

## 10. HONOUR YOUR HEALTH WITH GENTLE NUTRITION
Choose to eat food that honours both your health and your taste buds. Don't force yourself to drink spirulina smoothies if you don't like the taste (if you do, then go for it!); the food you eat should taste good and make you feel good. One snack, meal or day of eating doesn't automatically make you deficient in nutrients: remember that it's your overall food patterns that shape your health.

*Remember that these are principles, not commandments.*

Because it's not prescriptive: it's about realising that there's no 'right' or 'wrong' way to eat.

Aleeza summarises: 'Intuitive eating is a philosophy that rejects traditional dieting and instead encourages people to listen to their own body cues to decide when to eat, what to eat and how much to eat. This may sound like an impossible dream for some people, particularly if they have a history of dieting, because diets dictate what to eat, often resulting in people losing touch with their own hunger and satiety cues and food preferences.

'However, it is possible to get back in touch with one's body signals and learn how to eat intuitively, which will, ultimately, help to develop a healthy relationship with food. Instead of unhealthy behaviours that diet culture teaches, such as to ignore hunger and delay/skip meals, intuitive eating teaches one to honour one's hunger and to eat regularly. It also encourages one to see all foods as equal and no foods as off limits. Additionally, it empowers people to cope with their feelings without resorting to food. Given my specialism in eating disorders, I have seen thousands of patients who have ditched diet culture and learnt to become intuitive eaters, which has eliminated their fear of food, given them permission to eat what they want and allowed them to find true food freedom.'

Where to start? Aleeza suggests establishing a regular eating pattern – for me, as mentioned, this was three times a day, breakfast, lunch and dinner, with two snacks in between. 'This will help prevent you from becoming overly hungry at mealtimes, which risks bingeing and eating past fullness. Regular eating also helps hunger and satiety cues to becomes more reliable again.'

The second step is to acknowledge that all food groups play a role in helping the body function normally: some food groups help to keep blood sugar levels stable, like complex carbohydrates, which in turn prevents sugar cravings. Other food groups help to promote a feeling of fullness and satiety, like protein and fat, allowing people to feel satisfied for longer. 'I have seen thousands of patients who have embraced a balanced way of eating, which has helped them to feel more satisfied after meals and in control of their eating,' says Aleeza.

I have to interject here with something that I've been debating mentioning in this chapter but feel, ultimately, compelled to discuss: I, personally, feel that while there is a lot of talk about intuitive eating and listening to your body, particularly on Instagram, there is less discussion about where to begin with forming a healthy relationship with food. While I wanted to be an intuitive eater and listen to my body, I also wanted to know what and how much I should be eating. I wanted to strike the right balance, for me, between eating in order to nourish my body in the best possible way and eating the things I want to eat and enjoy food. It's all very well and good to read an Instagram post that says, 'Start listening to your body', but when you are totally disconnected from your body, have no idea what your body needs and have only very diet culture-skewed nutritional knowledge, that's difficult to do. (I knew that celery was a negative-calorie food but what nutrition did it actually bring to my body? I had no idea.) So learning about the role of each food group in our physiology was very beneficial as it helped me to understand why I needed each of them. A brief breakdown of each might help you, too.

The below is based on a model that Aleeza kindly shared with me:

**1. PROTEIN:** helps us maintain our muscle mass, skin and hair. Plus it's crucial for aiding any cellular and muscle-related recovery or daily performance. You can find protein in foods like meat, fish, eggs, dairy products, tofu and nuts.

**2. FAT:** a key element within a balanced diet, fat helps give your body energy, protects your organs, supports cell growth and is critical for the absorption of fat-soluble vitamins. You can find fats in foods like oily fish, avocado, cream, olives, mayonnaise, oily dressings and salad cream. Unsaturated fatty acids are types of fats found in foods like avocados, olives, olive oil and oily fish, whereas saturated fats tend to be found in butter, the fat in meat and the fat in cow's milk and other dairy. You want more unsaturated fat than saturated fat but all are fine in correct portions and proportions.

**3. FIBRE:** has lots of health benefits, including being associated with lower risk of heart disease, stroke, type-2 diabetes and bowel cancer. It also helps aid digestion and prevent constipation. Top tip: to ensure more fibre in your diet, stock your freezer up with frozen fruit and veg (frozen contains just as many nutrients as fresh fruit and veg) and eat the potato skin! If you're looking to increase your fibre, it's worth noting that wholegrain bread, cereals and pasta contain more than refined ones.

**4. CARBOHYDRATES:** these are your body's main source of energy. They help fuel your brain, kidneys, heart muscles and central nervous system. Wholegrain carbohydrates contain fibre that aids in digestion, helps you feel full and keeps blood cholesterol levels in check.

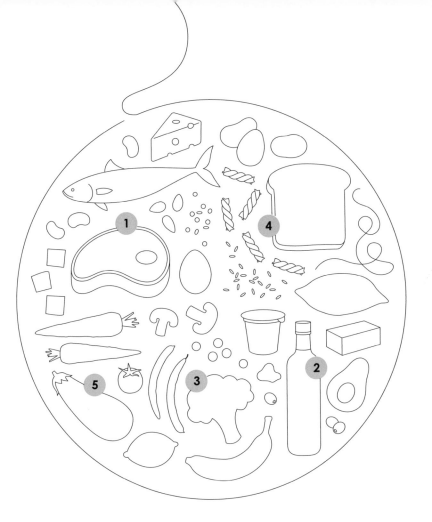

**5. FRUIT & VEGETABLES:** they contain important vitamins and minerals alongside providing the body with fibre.

**LOW-NUTRIENT FOOD** like chocolate, sweets, biscuits, cakes, crisps and ice cream: these are all things that most of us enjoy eating and there is nothing wrong with consuming them in moderation as part of a balanced diet.

'Assigning moral value to food threatens self-esteem and can cause people to feel ashamed and guilty about their eating habits, which can lead to dysfunctional eating or even an eating disorder.'

ALEEZA ROSENBERG

While it's important to learn about the different food groups and the function they play in the body, it's also vital to avoid labelling foods as 'good' or 'bad' – something which is very tied up in diet mentality. 'Food is not "good" or "bad" but so many people frequently talk about their behaviour value in relation to what kind of food they have been eating, thereby assigning a kind of moral value to food – even though it doesn't have any,' says Aleeza.

'The foods we eat, how much exercise we do or a number on the scale does not determine the value and worth we hold as human beings. We are worthy regardless of how we eat. Assigning moral value to food threatens self-esteem and can cause people to feel ashamed and guilty about their eating habits, which can lead to dysfunctional eating or even an eating disorder.'

It's difficult to combat this 'good/bad' dichotomy when it comes to food, particularly when it has been so ingrained in us by diet culture, but Aleeza advises working towards considering the nutrient value of food without giving it any moral value. 'It's absolutely OK to want chocolate or ice cream sometimes, just like it is OK to want fruit, vegetables and wholegrains.'

What about hunger and fullness cues – how can we wake them up? Once you've established a regular eating pattern, your body's physiology should be closer to working properly again and produce the necessary hunger and fullness hormones – but it's a case of identifying the certain symptoms that try to signal to us when we need to eat and when we need to stop eating. 'This often requires guidance and practice – particularly if one has been dieting for a long time or has been below their "set point" weight for a long period of time,' says Aleeza. 'Once a person knows what symptoms to look out for and can recognise when their body is hungry and when they are full, they are able to tune into these signals, which they can then use as a guide as to when to eat instead of following diet rules.

'Diet rules teach us to delay eating until ravenous, which is incredibly unhelpful – it risks blood sugars plummeting too low, which can trigger eating past fullness or bingeing. Waiting until you are extremely hungry or stopping eating only when you are uncomfortably full are two extremes – both of which should be avoided.'

Mindfulness was a huge help for me in becoming familiar with my hunger and fullness cues. Giving myself a second to check in with my body and using a hunger and fullness scale (see opposite) to determine how I was feeling allowed me, eventually, to be more in tune with my body.

This will help you tackle physical hunger but you may also need to do some work on emotional hunger – this is, of course, totally dependent on your individual situation. For me, this looked like finishing my meal, feeling full physically, but still feeling like I needed more.

'If you are still feeling physically hungry, give yourself permission to respond to that hunger by eating more,' says Aleeza. However, if you are persistently feeling like you need more even once full,

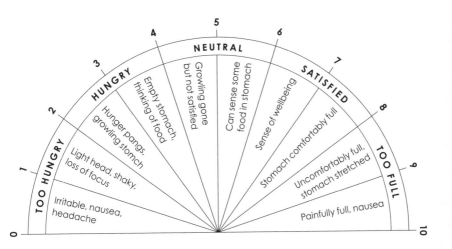

it could be that your emotional hunger needs a bit of attention. 'Many people use foods for emotional comfort, reward or to escape negative emotions. If one's goal is to achieve a healthy relationship with food, not only do you need to learn how to nourish your body by knowing when to eat, what to eat and how much to eat, but you also need to learn to recognise your emotional triggers to eating: these could be stress, anxiety or low mood. It might then be helpful to learn some alternative coping strategies to regulate these emotions in a way so that you don't need to resort to food. Sometimes, people struggle to recognise when they are feeling an emotion and what feeling it is, so I not only teach people how to tune into their physical cues of hunger and fullness, but also their emotions.'

Again, something else I found very difficult. Leaning into the uncomfortable emotions I was feeling, rather than quashing

'It is possible for everyone to develop a healthy relationship with food – even those who have been stuck in the diet cycle for many years or someone with an eating disorder.'

ALEEZA ROSENBERG

them with food, was painful. But useful in helping to uncover what was really going on with me.

I'm aware that I'm simplifying this process – and, again, I was lucky enough to have a therapist to guide me through this. I know how difficult and painful this can be and so I'd highly recommend seeking the advice of a dietitian if you can. If you can't, there are other books that really delve into the intuitive eating process, such as *Intuitive Eating: A Revolutionary Anti-Diet Approach* by Evelyn Tribole and Elyse Resch and *Just Eat It* by Laura Thomas.

And, while taking on all of these different steps, it's imperative that you approach the process with self-compassion. 'This is a long, difficult process – especially for people who have a history of dieting and in whom the diet mentality is ingrained. Dieting encourages habitual, unhealthy behaviours that are incongruent with intuitive eating: these habits are difficult to break and there is understandably the fear of adopting a new way of eating if one has relied on dieting to feel in control for so long.'

Aleeza likens switching to this new way of eating to learning a new language, where, if you are taught why the new language is a better way of communication and are guided through the fundamentals, the rest is just practice and confidence, and in no time you are speaking it fluently: 'With repetition and time, these new habits can become effortless, instinctive and sustainable, reinforced by the realisation of how much better you feel physically and mentally, how much more in control you are with food and how less afraid you are of food and social eating.'

Think maybe this isn't possible for you? I get it, I thought that, too. And sometimes women who are in their fifties or sixties believe that the diet mentality is too entrenched in their psyche to attempt another way of eating. But Aleeza assures us this isn't the case: 'It is possible for everyone to develop a healthy relationship with food – even those who have been stuck in the diet cycle for many years or someone with an eating disorder. As per the learning a new language analogy, sometimes you just need someone to support you through the journey, motivate you and give you the confidence to change, provide the foundations and cheer you on until it becomes instinctive.'

Finally, I wanted to ask Aleeza what she would recommend to anyone who is struggling with their food right now – what would her top-line advice be?

'If you are on a diet, please ditch it. Consider replacing it with these behaviours that will not only nourish your body but also help regulate your hunger/fullness cues and make you feel more in control of your eating.'

I keep coming back to the fact that it's hard, and that's not to discourage you from trying, but to keep things realistic. What I want you to know above all else is that it's so, so worth it.

*Healing my relationship with food changed my life – and you deserve that, too.*

# LET'S SUMMARISE

If you feel you are ready to take the first steps towards embracing a healthier relationship with food but are not sure where to start, this is what Aleeza advises:

- Eat regularly in the day, ensuring you have regular meals and in-between snacks so that you are eating something every three to four hours.

- Educate yourself about the function of foods, as every food group has a particular role in our body and none of them should be off limits.

- Learn what appropriate portions are for each of these food groups so that you get enough to nourish your body without needing to use diet rules like calorie counting.

- Keep a diary to be more aware of how you see and use food, which will help you to determine whether you are an emotional eater.

- Ask yourself whether you are doing a healthy amount of exercise. Exercise is beneficial for one's mood and energy levels, is a great stress release and aids sleep. However, if you are doing an excessive amount of exercise, feeling compelled to exercise or using exercise to give yourself permission to eat, then seek support.

# CHAPTER 10

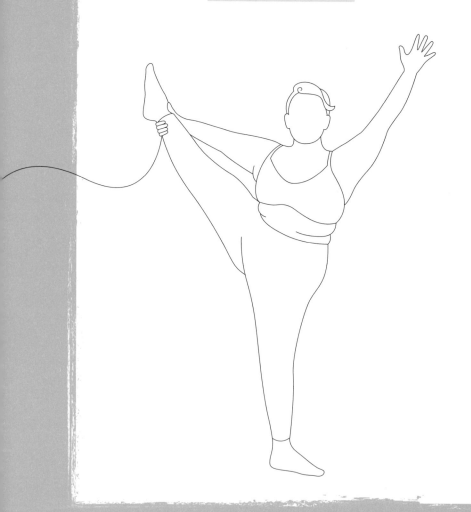

It's OK
to gain
weight

# Weight loss = good. Weight gain = bad. Right?

**Nope.**

That's certainly what we've been taught – idolise the skinny and condemn the fat – but weight gain, just like weight loss, is an inherent part of life. It occurs for many reasons: recovering from an eating disorder or disordered eating, mental health issues, stress, sleep issues, medication, physical illnesses, physical injuries, menopause, pregnancy and many more. Sometimes, it's for a simple or innocuous reason – maybe you changed jobs and no longer walk to work or maybe you are socialising more than you did before and are enjoying eating socially. Whatever the reason may be, weight fluctuations are a normal part of being a human and neither weight loss nor weight gain should be celebrated or villainised.

My weight gain was a result of recovering from an eating disorder and disordered eating. Many healthcare professionals, including dietitians and psychologists, state that we all have a set weight and body type, determined by genetics, environment and hormones, which is a certain range within which your body will settle and exist comfortably without us having to fight to stay there. I had always fought against my set point with dieting and restriction, so it took a while for my weight to level out – which it eventually did, largely due to relearning how to eat after a lifetime of listening to external sources from diet culture and picking up random rules that had ended up forming my eating patterns. There was also the interference of binge eating, which emerged as a totally normal biological response to my extended period of restriction.

The process was long and also painful. Incredibly painful because reaching my approximate set point required weight gain, and weight gain was something that I had feared practically above all else for my entire life. I was *terrified* of my body getting bigger, and I know I wasn't alone in this – many us are fearful of weight gain because we have been conditioned to believe that being fat is such a terrible thing.

While I was terrified about my body changing, I was also really desperate to recover from the internal prison of my eating disorder and I knew that meant ditching restriction and fostering a healthy relationship with food, which made weight gain a non-negotiable. But it was *hard*. Watching my body grow by the day impacted by mental health, which is not surprising: I was going against what I had spent practically my entire life trying to achieve.

I wasn't forced to get on the scales at my therapy session but I was strongly encouraged to do so and, as a perpetual people pleaser, I more than often ended up agreeing. I cannot describe the anguish of watching the numbers go up: I had dedicated years of my life – sacrificing relationships, career opportunities and happiness – to the painful, all-consuming struggle of forcing them down and this felt like I was suddenly at war with myself . . . and losing.

I've always leaned towards slightly baggier, more androgynous clothing but my wardrobe took on an entirely new aesthetic during that period: I wore jumpers that drowned my frame and wide-leg trousers to avoid any material clinging to my thighs. I even avoided social situations for fear of people noticing I had gained weight. I felt deeply ashamed and embarrassed; when I did see people, I felt the need to apologise to them about my weight gain . . . though I still don't understand why anyone would ever need to apologise to someone else for their weight fluctuation, or even explain it? It's so baffling and entirely unnecessary, obviously, but I know a lot of you will relate to this because women have long been taught to be apologetic about their bodies: I challenge you to recall a time when you went for a wax or a spray tan or a different kind of beauty treatment without apologising to the aesthetician.

I was starkly aware of the contrast between the comments I received when I thinner – 'You look amazing!', 'You're my body goals!', 'How do you stay so thin? I'm so jealous' and 'I wish I looked like you' are just a sample of the many compliments I received during my thinnest (and unhappiest!) phase – and the silence my new, bigger body was met with.

As I tried to become healthy, I was so consumed with fostering the negative feelings that it took a while for me to identify some of the benefits that weight gain can often bring with it. The more I worked on accepting my weight gain – and I have to point out again that I was lucky enough to be able to work with a psychologist throughout this – the more my eyes were opened to the good it had allowed into my life. What sticks out the most was the realisation that I was able to eat and eat regularly. I mentioned this previously but I have to reiterate what a huge relief this was after such a long period of being restrictive – I almost disbelieved that I was *allowed* to eat things I liked and so regularly . . . It felt euphoric, honestly (I'm hoping this book helps some of you get to that place, too). Armed with more energy and able to think more clearly – both because I was being nourished and also because I had more mental bandwidth without the constant, oppressive presence of the eating disorder – my work performance began to improve and I started to take pleasure in it once again. Restriction off the table, I also gained mental capacity for other things I previously hadn't been able to allocate any time to, like nurturing relationships with my family and my friends. With food rules ruling my life, I hadn't been the best person to be around: I was irritable, self-centred and too preoccupied to be present. Luckily, my friends, family and then-boyfriend understood what I had been through and afforded me compassion. On the aesthetic front, I also had a lot of hair regrowth – my hair was thinner than ever and in poor condition after years of malnutrition – and my skin shed its usual dullness for a slight glow.

My mum summed it up one day when she said: 'You've got your spark back. Before, you were just a shell of yourself.'

I acknowledge that this is specific to recovery from eating disorders and there are other reasons for weight gain that might not bring with it the same benefits. This is my story and my experience, but there are other benefits of weight gain, of course – it just very much depends on the individual and circumstance.

All of these advantages I experienced far, *far* outweighed any fleeting (it was always fleeting, no matter how long I tried to hold on to it) arbitrary pleasure I experienced from being a low weight; it just took me a while to see it. Which I acknowledge with compassion, given that we all grew up in a fatphobic culture that taught us that being thin was the best thing a human can achieve.

Armed with perspective and understanding of my weight gain process, I resolved to help other women who are struggling with weight gain. This came to a head during the pandemic when we were stripped of our normal routines and thrown into uncertain, unprecedented circumstances. Many people experienced weight gain and anxious feelings as a result. I spoke to lots of women who were even dreading lockdowns being lifted because it meant facing other people who might notice that they had put on weight. This stress was compounded by the diet industry, which – predictably – capitalised on this new, mass insecurity and ramped up its efforts to sell us weight loss solutions. The media and social media were more concerned with the 'Quarantine 15' – a term referring to pounds gained over the pandemic – and how to 'fix it quick', and fatphobic memes, than sharing mental health advice that could have *actually* been of benefit.

To counter all of the messages we hear from the media and diet culture about weight gain being **A VERY BAD THING** along with some of the panic around lockdown weight gain, I decided to share a series of posts depicting my own weight gain with the message: 'It's OK to gain weight.' It's a simple message and one that should be totally implicit, but because of the way we frame weight gain, this is actually a revolutionary stance. Many of the posts went viral and women from all over the world wrote to me expressing their relief at seeing this 'permission' being granted to them. Many had never even contemplated the idea that it's OK to gain weight. It's sad, isn't it?

Sad, but not surprising given that the way society tends to treat weight gain in other people is usually derogatory. Common narratives that accompany weight gain is:

- They've given up.

- They've let themselves go.

- They've thrown the towel in.

- They don't care about their appearance anymore.

- They've lost self-control.

One person actually did DM me after an 'It's OK to gain weight' post to tell me: 'You've really let yourself go.' I replied and told him that yes, I had, in fact, let myself go. I had let myself go and let myself *live*, and it was the most powerful thing I have ever done for myself. Weight gain

I had let myself go
and let myself *live*,
and it was the most
powerful thing
I have ever done
for myself.

was the external proof of this and I was damn proud of it. He responded with: 'OK but ur still ugly'.

Needless to say, I left it there.

There is so much power in reclaiming your weight gain and owning your own narrative and story. Even though this requires coming to terms with it, which, I know, can be hard. To help you, here are the things that aided me in my journey:

- **Turn to self-compassion.** It's OK to be struggling with weight gain and pushing those feelings down by pretending to yourself that it isn't challenging can make it even more difficult in the long term. Allow yourself to grieve your previous body or your fantasy of yourself at a lower weight. Grieve for it and gradually let go.

- **Think about the relationship you currently have with the scales.** Is weighing yourself doing you any good? Or is it causing you harm? I predict that it's likely the latter, given the power the scales have over so many of us when it comes to dictating our self-worth and taking away our inherent power as a human being. Consider re-evaluating your relationship with the scales and focusing instead on getting in tune with your body. Bear in mind, also, that the weight references you go off are likely put in place by arbitrary markers of health (like the BMI scale and the weight you were when you were a younger age).

- **Diversify your feed.** We'll dive into this at length in Chapter 13, along with a potential list of people to follow, but for now, know that it's a really vital step. Rid your feed of the thin ideal imagery that's rampant on social media and follow people who look like you and people that don't. Open your eyes up to new ideals and visions of beauty.

- **Focus on how you feel.** It's easy to focus on the reflection in the mirror or the number on the scale and let it affect you but this is only serving to relinquish power to diet culture. Reclaim the power by getting in touch with your body: for me, that's through exercise. I do a boxing or spin class and escape my own head for a while, focusing on what my body can *do*, rather than how it looks. I find this incredibly effective at shifting my mindset and making space for gratitude for my body. Another technique I used – and still do, in fact – was to complete a 'compassionate body scan' – you can find one on YouTube. It's an audio exercise that involves a guide moving your attention gently from your feet to your head and is intended to bring awareness to the myriad of sensations that occur throughout the body while offering gratitude and compassion, ultimately allowing for a greater sense of comfort. It is almost instantly effective at making me feel more at peace in my body.

- **Think about a new wardrobe.** I know this isn't possible for everyone – whether it's for financial reasons or due to the fact that many fat women aren't easily able to find clothes that fit at reasonable prices – but if you can, it will make a huge difference, even if you just purchase three or four new key pieces that you can rotate.

It's utterly demoralising to be confronted with a wardrobe full of clothes that no longer fit. You don't need the constant reminder, so be brave and either stash those clothes away where you can't see them, give them to a friend or charity or participate in a clothes swap for items your size. Whatever you do, please consider not squeezing yourself into clothes that don't fit: this is a crystal clear message to your body that it doesn't deserve comfort and it absolutely does.

- **Pay attention to your wardrobe.** OK so you've done a cull and now you're filling up your wardrobe with new clothes – make sure these clothes aren't merely props to hide your body. Look for things you like, that you feel good in and that you enjoy wearing. Swamping your body in clothes that don't threaten to reveal it is a way of allowing shame to dominate. Of course, you may have a preference for oversized clothing and there's nothing wrong with that! But make sure it's a style preference rather than a compulsion to hide your body.

- **Don't glamorise your old body.** This is especially relevant to people who have recovered from an eating disorder or disordered eating – it's easy to forget what was going on during the period of having a thinner body. Remember why it was important that you moved on from that.

- **Acknowledge that bodies change.** If your weight gain is due to another reason, remember that that is absolutely OK, too. Bodies fluctuate, it's part of being a human being and it's only because of the world we live in that weight loss is considered good and weight gain as bad.

- **Rid yourself of shame.** Your body changing does not deserve any kind of shame, that is an entirely negative emotion that brings no benefit. It needs to go and, as Christiane Northrup's famous quote goes: 'Shame cannot exist in the light.' So bring it into the light and open up to people you love and trust. I'm certainly not recommending you copy me and apologise to anyone and everyone for your weight gain but speaking about it in situations where you feel you can do so can be hugely helpful for offloading and also getting closer to acceptance.

- **Set boundaries with people immersed in diet culture.** Be super-aware of exactly what you do and don't need right now, and don't be scared to set your boundaries with people who are engaging in diet/weight talk and making you feel inadequate.

- **Try to gain perspective.** I struggled with how to word this one because I don't want to minimise your pain in any way. But gaining perspective was very helpful for me – identifying the things that I was grateful for in my life allowed me to expand my tunnel vision and focus on other, more important areas of my life. I know this is easier said than done but gratitude journaling really is helpful for gaining perspective.

'Shame cannot
exist in the light.'

CHRISTIANE NORTHRUP

- **Live your life.** Please don't cancel plans or avoid social occasions because of your weight gain. It's a cliché but it's true: you have one life and it's far too short to spend it holed up in your home because you're worrying about what people think about your body. You're treating yourself with shame and I guarantee you it won't make you feel any better.

- **Nourish your body.** This is incredibly important – lean into reconnecting with your body and its hunger and fullness cues and try to practise intuitive eating. Your body deserves to be nourished and treated well, no matter what size.

- **Is there a silver lining?** Consider if there have been any positive outcomes of your weight gain. For example, if your weight gain is a result of giving up restriction, it will be helpful to list your 'reasons to recover' (a better relationship with food, food freedom, more energy, more mental clarity, a better worklife and a better social life might be some of the benefits).

- **Educate yourself about fatphobia.** Revisit Chapter six, if you need to. Fatphobia is the reason we're so deeply uncomfortable with weight gain, so learning about it and tackling it will help to bring more peace with your own body.

- **Remember that weight gain isn't inherently bad.** Diet culture has done a number on us with regards to this belief but weight gain is not a bad thing; it's most definitely not a terrible failure, it's just a normal part of being a human. We can't forget the role that the patriarchy has to play in this, too – notice how weight gain for men is much more accepted and less judged?

- **Be patient with yourself.** Body acceptance takes time and patience. Understand that you're not going to feel great about your body overnight and make peace with the journey.

- **Get professional help if you need it.** If weight gain is seriously impacting your life, the best thing you can do for yourself is get some help. I am very aware that therapy isn't a possibility for everyone but if you are able to seek professional help in some capacity, I hugely recommend it.

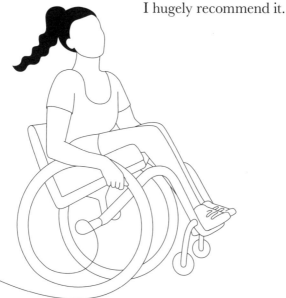

**Know that you are way more than your body.** You are so much more than a number on the scales or a dress size. The good, important stuff about you does not lie with the external, therefore it shouldn't actually matter what your body looks like and whether you've lost or gained weight. That undermines all the amazing things about us as individuals. The people around you still love you no matter your shape or size – and if they don't, that is categorically a *them* problem, NOT a *you* problem.

While these are all healthy things that you can put in place to prompt and accelerate your acceptance journey, there are some no-nos that you should try to avoid at all costs if you're struggling with weight gain:

**Don't panic.** Panic is futile – it's not a positive emotion and leaning into it can encourage punishing behaviour, which will lead you into dangerous territory.

**Don't do a fad diet.** I know it can feel tempting in the moment but, as we've explored at length, diets don't work. If you do lose weight, it's likely to come back – and possibly more so.

**Don't skip meals.** Again, it's tempting to skip meals when you're reeling from the shock of weight gain but this only causes you problems like destabilising your blood sugar and encouraging binge eating. Try to plan out your meals ahead of time to keep you feeling secure and stable.

- **Don't limit certain foods.** I used to restrict carbs when I noticed weight gain – I thought this was the fastest way of shedding the pounds but all it did was make me obsessed with carbs because I wasn't allowed them.

- **Don't punish yourself.** As we know, shame is not a positive emotion and standing in front of yourself in the mirror and calling yourself harsh words will not benefit you in any way. If you find yourself doing this, bring yourself back to a place of compassion.

- **Don't overexercise.** By all means, stick to your normal exercise regime but don't ramp it up in an attempt to lose the weight gained – this may lead to an unhealthy relationship with exercise and potentially harm your body.

- **Acknowledge and deal with feeling less 'attractive'.** If you're struggling with feeling less attractive after weight gain – because diet cultures deems thinness to be attractive and fatness to be ugly, of course – know that it's OK. It's important to acknowledge how you feel. But it's also important to remember that, firstly, nobody is scrutinising you as much as you. People might not even notice any weight gain – and if they do, why should that make you less attractive to them? What makes people *truly* attractive is not how they look. That's not a platitude, that's a cold, hard fact. And if they *are* judging you, maybe it's time to question if they're even worthy of your time and energy.

Even if you're putting all of this into practice, there are certain things that can pop up and derail us. For me, that was seeing past pictures of myself when I was thinner. I struggled with longing for that body and feeling like I was stuck in a rut of comparing my current self to my old self. I know that's a huge problem for many of you, too, especially with constant Facebook and Instagram reminders of old photos – I receive messages daily from women who have been getting to grips with their new body and are suddenly triggered by past pictures. I get it – god knows I've been there. Please bookmark this chapter so that whenever this happens to you, you can come back and read the advice all over again. If it's something that pops up regularly, you can block memories on Facebook.

Another thing that can be hugely triggering is reactions from other people. More often than not, these reactions actually live in our heads, rather than in real life. We're scared of what people might think of our weight gain, or that they might gossip about it to others, and those thoughts can be debilitating.

When I first started to gain weight, I sobbed to my therapist about this: I couldn't bear the idea of people talking about my weight behind my back. I will never forget the two words she said to me that helped to entirely change my perspective on this: 'So what?' I floundered – I honestly didn't know how to respond. I didn't actually know why this would be such a big deal and I couldn't work it out. The thoughts weren't immediately alleviated by her words but they definitely sowed a seed of doubt: does it *really* matter if people notice I've gained weight? I was no longer sure. Eventually, I worked out that no, it really doesn't matter. Because what other people think of me has nothing to do with me – it doesn't, and shouldn't, impact my life. Someone spots my weight gain – then what? They might say to someone else, 'Hasn't she put on weight?' – then what? The world keeps turning, right?! They continue to live their life and I continue to live mine. It doesn't actually mean anything.

Something else to consider very seriously is that people are often way too wrapped in their own lives and insecurities to care. Yes, they might notice your weight gain (they also might not!) but they are too involved in themselves to do anything *but* notice . . . If they do and they are one of those people who comment on other people's weight, then I must reiterate that it's on them, not you. It is almost certainly a huge indication of their own internal pressures and struggles with body image – that doesn't make it right, but it's true. Feel sorry for them that they're living with these unresolved issues but don't let them be projected onto you.

OK, wow. That's a lot of info and a lot of advice, I know. I poured everything I could into this chapter because I have been there, I get it and I want to provide you with some relief and an alternative to the feelings of shame and disappointment that weight gain can bring with it. I hope I don't sound like I'm preaching because I know all too well just how hard this can be. There were a lot of ups and downs and backwards and forwards for me before I could accept my new body – a lot of this advice I had a really hard time putting into practice. Especially the compassion, which is the vital component that underpins all of this. But it is so imperative, and so if there's just one thing that you take away with you from this chapter,

let it be that. Your body has got you through your life so far
– that is something to be celebrated. It doesn't deserve to be
treated with disgust, shame and hatred. You need to treat your
body gently; you deserve nothing but kindness.

*And remember this: taking up space is allowed. You do not need to be the smallest version of yourself to be accepted.*

Now read that again.

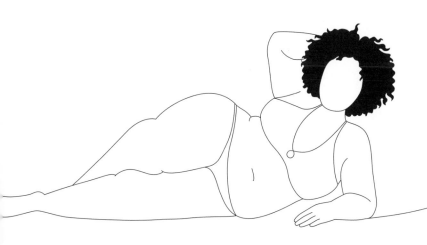

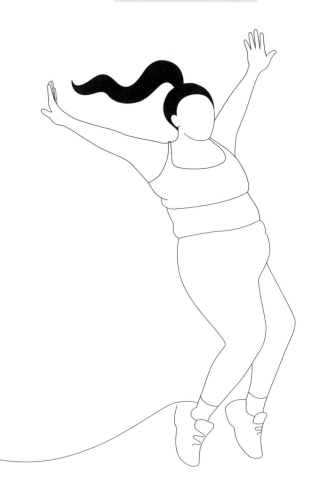

CHAPTER 11

Fitness does not equate to thinness

# Exercise has always been incredibly complicated for me.

From the moment I understood that it can affect weight, it has been inextricably tied to how my body looks.

At around the age of 14, I found a book in the library that recommended exercises for a flat stomach. I took it home and spent every night for the next month working my way through the crunches and leg raises, excited to wake up one morning and see a perfectly flat stomach. Of course, that didn't happen – despite the advice frequently offered in magazines, via Google and even by health professionals, you can't exercise your way to a flat tummy – so I moved on to holding a plank for ten minutes every day as I read *that* was the best way to tone your core. Though I soon realised that it didn't seem to be having an effect on how I looked in the mirror, so I moved on to something else . . .

And this is how my relationship with exercise continued for the next 15 or so years: throw myself into a new type of regime, go hell for leather for a month or so, then revert back to doing no exercise and pledging to stick to controlling my food intake instead. You name it, I tried it: running, spinning, dancing, swimming, squash, weightlifting, pilates, yoga and circuit-training at various different studios.

I even did a week-long bootcamp when I was 22. It was the most physically gruelling week of my life. I consumed around 1,000 calories a day, while my fellow bootcampers and I spent from 7am to 4pm doing various kinds of intense exercise, including running, circuit training, boxing and hiking. I distinctly remember a girl being shouted at to continue doing burpees while she was retching or 'the group will pay!' It was as hellish as it sounds. But the thought of weight loss – that was not needed in any way, I was already at a low weight for me – kept me going.

I lost weight, got home and booked into circuit-training five days a week as I was terrified of gaining the weight back. But five days of demanding exercise that I didn't actually enjoy each week wasn't sustainable – and, I believe, as a non-expert, not healthy, either – and that soon fell by the wayside.

As well as a means to manipulate my weight, I used exercise as a punishment for eating too much. If I went over my entirely self-imposed calorie limit, I turned to exercise as a means to appease the anger I felt at myself for the 'overconsumption'. It was incredibly disordered – but I suspect a lot of this might be resonating with quite a few of you . . .

But . . . why? Why are some of us in this disordered space with exercise? I spoke to Tally Rye, an intuitive and health-first fitness coach, to explore this.

'As children, moving our body was about play, adventure and fun with our friends. But for many of us growing up, that soon evolved into rigid forms of exercise becoming punishment and penance for enjoying food, as well as being a way to control our bodies and appearance to fit society's beauty and body standards,' she says.

Essentially, what once felt joyful and free becomes burdened with rules and rigidity, with new meaning: control your appearance. All introduced, of course, by diet culture. By the idea that we have to look a certain way (thin) and conform to a narrow standard of beauty. The fitness industry capitalises on this, tapping into diet culture by marketing their products by dangling the promise of body transformations – you know, the classic 'before and after' – and promises of shifting pounds and 'getting into shape'. (Sidenote: you're already in shape. What is 'in shape'? In what shape?) Exercise is no longer about enjoying moving your body, it's about changing your body, and the considerable non-appearance-related benefits of fitness are largely ignored.

Through the toxic combination of diet culture and the fitness industry, fitness becomes equated to thinness. The use of transformation pictures in particular serves to reinforce this: the after picture never shows a person who has gained weight, right? They're always in a noticeably smaller body, perpetuating the (false) narrative that you have to be thin to be fit, and that getting fit is about getting thin. But, as Tally points out, 'these are two entirely different pursuits'. Changes in fitness levels are rarely referred to in transformation stories and, if they are, they come secondary to the amount of weight lost. In a culture obsessed with weight, I don't think any of this is surprising, but isn't it so incredibly toxic?

Until a few years ago, I don't think I could have listed any other reasons (maybe outside of 'good for your heart') to exercise apart from weight loss. How many can you think of? There are so, so many – they're just not talked about enough. Here are some to get us thinking:

- **Improved mood and wellbeing.** When we exercise, our body releases chemicals called endorphins, which trigger a positive feeling in the body. Exercise has been shown to improve mood and decrease feelings of depression, anxiety and stress as well as increase our self-esteem.

- **Improved brain cognition.** By increasing your heart rate, exercise promotes the flow of blood and oxygen to your brain, aiding brain health and memory and protecting mental function among older adults.

- **Muscle benefits.** Muscle-strengthening activities like lifting weights can help increase or maintain mass and strength, which can help especially with older adults as reduced muscle mass and muscle strength can become a problem as we age.

- **Bone benefits.** Exercise works on bones as it does on muscles, making them stronger. When we're younger, exercise is important for building bones and when we're older, it's essential for maintaining bone strength. When you exercise regularly and consume sufficient nutrients, your bone adapts by building more bone and becoming denser. Two million people in the UK have osteoporosis, and women are at much higher risk. Exercising regularly throughout our lives is one way we can guard against this.

- **Increased energy levels.** Moving more can help give you energy through several mechanisms, including boosting oxygen circulation inside your body.

- **Sleep aid.** Regular exercise has been proven to help you relax and sleep better, as well as alleviating daytime sleepiness.

- **Reduced risk of chronic disease.** Regular exercise has been shown to improve insulin sensitivity and heart health, as well as decrease blood pressure and cholesterol levels.

- **Contributes to skin health.** Moderate exercise is found to provide antioxidant protection and promote blood flow, which can protect your skin and contribute to overall skin health.

- **Boosts sex drive.** Studies consistently show that exercise equals a higher sex drive and better sexual function.

But it's important to know that to get many of these benefits, we don't need to do strenuous, vigorous exercise. You don't need to go out and buy a lycra all-in-one, complete five HIIT sessions in a week and not be able to move for another week after that: just getting up and moving and raising your heart rate is good for you. According to the NHS, adults aged 19 to 64 should do at least two and a half hours of aerobic exercise a week – but this includes just walking somewhere at a decent pace.

So why do we believe that 'if it doesn't challenge you, it doesn't change you' (to quote a famous fitness industry saying)? Diet culture, of course. 'Diet culture tells us that exercise is simply a means to an end for weight loss and body manipulation, that it is just a tool to control the body – therefore, the goal is to earn and burn food, and calories become the focus,' says Tally Rye. So much of the diet and fitness industries' messaging sends a clear signal: exercise is not something to enjoy, rather something to endure, with the goal of losing weight.

There are countless past examples from pop culture that have reinforced a toxic take on exercise – and, unfortunately, we're not much further on now. In 2020, the BBC aired a show called *The Restaurant That Burns Off Calories*. Hosted by a maitre d' and a doctor, the show saw 20 people eat lunch in a restaurant before revealing that there was a gym attached, where 25 others were working out on exercise bikes, treadmills and rowing machines to 'burn off' the calories consumed by the diners. The show was met with backlash and UK eating disorder charity BEAT publicly condemned it. 'We know that the myth that all calories eaten must be cancelled out through exercise has the potential to be devastating to those suffering from or vulnerable to eating disorders,' BEAT's director of services, Caroline Price, said in a statement. 'Being told how much activity it would take to burn off particular food risks triggering the illness further and we strongly advise anyone at risk to avoid these sources of information.' While the show was incredibly damaging for people with eating disorders, it also served to reinforce the diet culture view of exercise as simply a way of burning calories and counteracting food consumption.

Unpicking all of
the deconditioning
we have experienced –
with diet culture, body
image and exercise –
is not an overnight task.

I am someone who is still working on their own relationship with exercise and I think it might still take me a while yet. Given my focus has been on eating and nourishment during my recovery from eating disorders, exercise has had to take a back seat. So while I know that all the advice in this chapter is accurate and what I should be practising myself, I do feel a *bit* like a fraud as I write this! I'll get there, though.

But my attitude to and feelings around exercise *have* vastly improved from the days when I would jump from one unsustainable regime to the next in order to find something that changed my body. Rather than seeing exercise as something to be carried out with the sole purpose of altering my appearance, I have transitioned to a place where I do it because I know that it's a positive thing to do – for both my physical and mental health. Don't get me wrong, sometimes I'm not overly excited about working out but I appreciate what it does for me and I know that my mood is boosted as a result.

Detangling exercise from weight loss for me was difficult. Even when I thought I was managing to separate the two, I realised old thoughts crept in. It's a process. Unpicking all of the deconditioning we have experienced – with diet culture, body image and exercise – is not an overnight task. It's something we have to work at, and that's OK. Every so often, I still have some involuntary, disordered thoughts arise when it comes to my fitness – for example, when I'm in a class, I might become tempted to push past my body's limits or I might find myself thinking about doing a class the day after eating a heavy meal – but I'm able to identify them and compassionately encourage myself to enter a more rational, conscious mode, and I believe that's what matters.

# DO YOU HAVE A HEALTHY RELATIONSHIP WITH EXERCISE?

You might automatically answer 'yes' but because fitness and diet culture are so entwined, many of us have a disordered relationship with movement without even realising it – and I suspect that many of you reading this following section might be surprised by the potential red flags to look out for:

**DO YOU EXERCISE TO COMPENSATE FOR CALORIES CONSUMED?** For example, have you ever been for a run purely because you had a big meal or 'too many carbs' the night before and you feel, on some level, that you have to 'make up' for it? Nourishing your body is not something to be punished. An obsession with attempting to burn off your food through exercise can be classed as a form of bulimia, called non-purging type bulimia.

**ARE YOU TRYING TO CHANGE SPECIFIC BODY PARTS?** Maybe you are fixated on having a flat stomach or your workouts are mainly based around toning your thighs and bum. This indicates a potential problem with body image, as a preoccupation with how you look is not healthy physically or mentally, and countless hours exercising won't fix your body image.

**DO YOU SOMETIMES FEEL GUILT OR ANXIETY WHEN YOU MISS A WORKOUT?** Exercise should be a tool to improve our mental health, not worsen it.

Finding an exercise I actually enjoyed doing was pivotal for me. I always thought I liked circuit-training but I think that, actually, I'd just heard that it was meant to burn a lot of calories. I used to make myself run but I really despise the monotony of running. So I went through a period of trying different kinds of exercises to see what genuinely appealed to me.

I settled on spinning classes and boxing. I've always loved boxing, so I bought myself a course of classes, a boxing bag and some gloves. And now it's an activity I look forward to doing. I also really enjoy spinning classes – I love the fun, high energy aspect – and so I try to fit in one session of each in per week. Sometimes I don't – at the moment, I am incredibly busy writing this book so I haven't done anything for a couple of weeks, and that's absolutely OK. I am compassionate and patient with myself, and I'm only going to do what feels right for me.

I encourage you, too, to reflect on what you think you might enjoy and what makes you feel good when it comes to exercise – whether this is exercising with friends, exercising in a group, listening to music or podcasts as you exercise, being outdoors or playing sport. And afford yourself time and patience – if you've spent your entire life hating exercise and treating it as punishment, it's going to be a big adjustment.

Which leads me to intensity of exercise. Instead of punishing myself in gruelling workouts that left me exhausted (because I thought that was best for weight loss), I decided to listen to my body and let it lead me. If I go to a spin class and I'm hyped and feeling super-energetic, I'll try to keep up with the instructor. But if I go and realise that I'm just feeling like I want to take it a bit easier, I go at my own pace. I know now that I am not a 'failure' if I try but decide I'm just not up for it, or if I don't do what I'd set out to do. There are many factors at play when it comes to how active we might be feeling, like hormones and mental health, and staying connected to and honouring my body is so important and a real marker of success for me.

That's my story, but I wanted a guide to fostering a better relationship with exercise from an expert, so I asked Tally Rye, a pioneer of intuitive movement. Intuitive movement, she explains, is a framework to help people strip back and re-assess their relationship with exercise so they can move away from diet culture and rebuild and reclaim trust and connection with themselves, so that movement becomes a positive and joyful experience.

Here are the nine principles of intuitive movement, as outlined in Rye's book *Train Happy*:

**1. REJECT THE DIET MENTALITY.** 'This is about shifting the intention behind movement and finding your own intrinsic motivation to move. Start by acknowledging the negative impact that weight-centric fitness has had and making a conscious decision for movement to become about joy, self-care, community and a fun physical challenge,' writes Rye. She recommends curating your social media to reflect this, unfollowing the diet culture #fitspos and instead following diverse accounts that show joyful movement in a variety of ways and by a variety of people: @meg.boggs,

@kanoagreene, @jonelleyoga, @missfitsworkout, @sophjbutler and @fatgirlshiking are a few suggestions to get you started. Following these brilliant creators will not only help shift your mindset from seeing exercise as something that belongs only to a thin, non-disabled participant to anyone who is interested in exercise, but it also helps to re-establish the joy in movement away from any kind of disordered control. 'This is an opportunity to think about ditching the diet culture tools, including taking a break from fitness watches and stopping progress pictures, scales and measurements.'

**2. HONOUR YOUR EXERCISE APPETITE.** Just like with intuitive eating, this is about building awareness of your body's appetite both for movement and for rest. 'If you're not sure where to start with this, these questions may help:

- How would you like to move your body?
- How energetic do you feel today?
- When do you want to move? What time of day feels best?
- How long do you want to exercise for?
- When is your body asking for rest? What are those signals?

Listening to your body's answers to the questions above means that you can begin to engage in exercise on your *own* terms. By honouring your body's needs for rest and movement, you will strengthen the trust and signals will become increasingly clear.'

*This all seems so . . . simple, and obvious, right?!*

Yet we so often push ourselves to override our body's signals in the pursuit of manipulating our weight. Reconnecting to your body feels magical after not allowing it to have a say for so long.

**3. GIVE YOURSELF UNCONDITIONAL PERMISSION TO REST.** We've been, unfortunately, conditioned by diet culture to fear rest and feel guilty about not moving our bodies. 'But rest is a crucial element of a sustainable and healthy relationship with exercise. This principle is about reframing rest and challenging the inner dialogue that tells us its "wrong" or "lazy" or "going to undo all your hard work".'

You can tackle this by giving yourself repeated permission to rest. It may well feel challenging and uncomfortable but it is vital. You may believe that if you let yourself rest then you will never voluntarily do exercise again, but in reality, honouring rest helps to create a sense of safety and trust that ultimately allows you to explore movement in a way that feels good for you, at your own pace and only when you're ready.

**4. MAKE PEACE WITH EXERCISE.** 'In the same way diet culture taught us to have "good" and "bad" foods, it did the same with fitness,' says Rye. 'For example, many of us think that super sweaty cardio workouts are "good" because of the underlying narrative that "good" exercise is about calorie burn, and low intensity workouts like yoga are "bad" because they don't exhaust the body in the same way.'

But here's the thing: neither is better than the other as all forms of movement have their own function and their own place in our routines. Rather than how many calories it burns, it's instead about the intention behind the workout and, as we shift to a place of movement for self-care, that will inform the exercise choices we ultimately make. For me, honouring this principle meant ditching HIIT training. If you like it, that's great – but let's just say it is not the exercise for me! The constant 'am I going to vomit?' uncertainty never really made the workout pleasant.

**5. CHALLENGE THE FITNESS POLICE.** Many of us have created a set of rules around exercise – again, thank you diet culture! 'Perhaps you have to work out for a certain amount of time and intensity? Or you must complete a certain number of sessions a week and never miss a Monday? Ask yourself where these rules came from and how do they make you feel about exercise. Probably not great, right? So challenge them. For example, you may have previously told yourself you "must" work out for 60 minutes in the gym but actually you realise you feel satisfied with shorter workouts that last 20–30 minutes. So honour that and do what feels best for you.'

I remember thinking that if the workout didn't last very long, it just wasn't worth doing. And so, I would push myself to reach a certain amount of time, despite my body being quite unwilling to cooperate. This, of course, not only meant that I was ignoring my body, but it also contributed to cementing exercise as something to be endured, rather than enjoyed.

**6. DISCOVER THE FEEL-GOOD FACTOR.** 'Exercise is *not* a form of punishment and should never be motivated by guilt and shame,' says Rye. 'Instead, approach movement as a form of self-care, self-respect and self-expression. Focus on how good your chosen activities make you feel – proud, strong, confident, powerful, connected to yourself and part of a community.' I found that, for me, reframing exercise as part of my self-care routine was powerful – seeing it as something I make time to do for me and me only, to keep me feeling my best mentally, was a really positive shift.

**7. LEARN HOW IT CAN HELP YOU TO MANAGE EMOTIONS.** 'Movement can be a therapeutic tool to help us build inner strength and resilience so we can dig deeper into our feelings and emotions,' says Rye. It is, of course, not to be used in place of therapy or medication, but it is a powerful supporting tool alongside. This can include slowing down on sad days and connecting with emotion through a yoga sequence (I'm not entirely sure yoga is for me – I think I'm too impatient and in need of constant stimulation so I find it a little slow, BUT I know that it has a hugely positive impact on so, so many people) putting boxing gloves on and punching out the stress (definitely more my vibe!) or getting outside in nature to get perspective on life. Often we use exercise as a means to avoid emotions but an intuitive approach is about acknowledging and working with them. And I don't know about you, but any other ways of managing my often-overwhelming emotions is always welcome!

**8. ACCEPT YOUR BODY AS IT IS NOW.** As I hope we've all agreed by now, your body is not a 'before' waiting for an 'after'. You do not have to weigh less before you are 'allowed' to move your body. 'Fitness is not just reserved for thin people – it can and should be for everyone, which you will see reflected in the Instagram accounts I've previously recommended. As we start to accept our bodies, we stop fighting them and learn to work *with* them, with respect, kindness and compassion.'

This feels like a good time to touch on *that* Nike plus-size mannequin furore. In 2019, the activewear brand unveiled a line-up of plus-size mannequins at its flagship London store and while the move was hailed as a hugely positive step for inclusivity, it also prompted criticism. One journalist wrote an article for a very well-known newspaper entitled, 'Obese mannequins are selling a dangerous lie'. The criticism was heavy for many who had felt empowered by the inclusion of the plus-size mannequins, but it was, hopefully, overpowered by the hundreds if not thousands of people who condemned the backlash. The journalist eventually wrote an apology. Because every single body deserves not just normal clothes, but gym clothes, too – because every single body deserves movement, if this is a possibility.

## 9. HAVE A HEALTHY RELATIONSHIP WITH GOALS.

When you strip your relationship with exercise back to basics in order to cultivate an intuitive approach, you may take a necessary break from structure and goals, which is encouraged. However, when you are exercising in harmony with your body's needs and feeling good about working out, you may want to set certain goals that you would like to achieve, such as running a half marathon, and for this, you will need to add guidance and structure back in. However, we are still being gentle with ourselves because our targets and what we do to reach them are no longer rigid; we allow room for flexibility and options for extra rest, incorporate movement we enjoy and ultimately listen to our body first and the training plan second. 'It can be really cool and motivating to have a goal to work towards but we are now flexible in our approach,' says Rye. (Side note: you don't have to work towards goals if you don't want to!)

I remember when I first read Tally's book and I was kind of blown away by these principles. They make so much sense but exercise had never, ever been presented to me in this way before. And I think the advice that underpins all of them is compassion – something I didn't feel had ever been encouraged in movement before. But employing self-compassion is so powerful and so liberating. It takes the pressure off and allows you to connect with your own body . . . Which is what this book is all about.

I know that there's a chance that you're feeling a bit lost right now: either because you don't do any exercise at all and don't know where to start or you have realised your relationship with exercise is actually not very healthy. But be very kind to yourself and take it step by step. Assess where you are right now, have compassion for that – it's not your fault you don't have a good relationship with exercise – and try to reframe how you feel about movement. Get curious about different ways to move your body and get exploring! Most of it won't stick – it didn't for me – BUT you may well find something that you genuinely love.

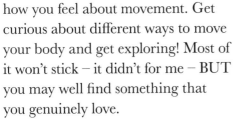

# CHAPTER 12

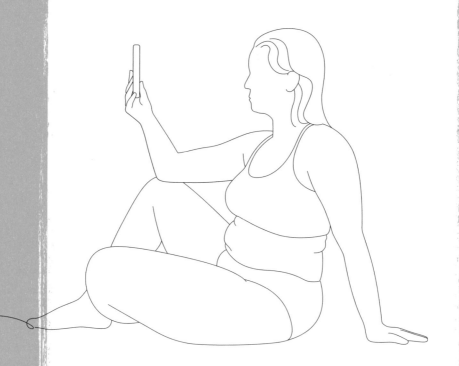

# Deconditioning is powerful

I was going to start this chapter by saying 'we are what we consume'...

But then I realised what it reminded me of – that trite phrase we've all heard coming from diet culture, 'You are what you eat.'

It's often bandied about, designed to induce shame around eating choices, and it isn't true – obviously. If you eat a biscuit, you don't become a biscuit. It's stupid.

But what is true is that what we eat does affect our health, energy levels and wellbeing. For example, if you eat hardly any vegetables, you will probably struggle to give your body all the vitamins it needs. Similarly, you are not defined by who you choose to follow and interact with on social media but it *can* have a big influence on our mental health and self-esteem. The average person in the UK spends 109 minutes per day on social media – nearly two hours.[34] So it's bound to have an impact on how we see ourselves and we know it causes body dissatisfaction: so much so, that I've dedicated an entire chapter to exploring it. In fact, scientist Clarissa Silva conducted studies in 2017 that showed that 60 per cent of people using social media believe it has a negative impact on their self-esteem. When you look at it like this, I think it becomes quite clear that actively controlling which social media feeds you let into your life and asking yourself how they make you feel is an important part of combatting diet culture and improving your relationship with your own body.

But first let's ask . . . why? Why does social media impact our self-esteem? And why do we keep going back to it, refreshing our feeds, even when we know that we're not always using it in a way that's enjoyable or healthy?

I think it's important to lay out, firstly, just how entwined social media is with our daily lives: the average person aged 25–34 in the UK spends 137 minutes on social media per day, while globally, the average for that age group is 157 minutes.[34] It accounts for a huge part of our day and, specifically, a huge part of the messaging that we consume in a day and often internalise. It doesn't look like this is going to be reducing any time soon – if anything, our usage is only going to increase.

Social media relies predominantly on visuals, which is where the harm comes in. This visual nature reinforces the idea that our validation lies with how we look and encourages self-objectification, which is when we place the importance of our bodies on how it looks, rather than its function, and view our worth as something that can be judged based on our appearance.

Comparison also has a huge part to play. As we discussed in Chapter nine, humans are hardwired to compare and 88 per cent of women admitted to comparing themselves to images in the media, with half saying the comparison is unfavourable,[35] while a 2011 experiment revealed that 'people who look at attractive users [on Facebook] have fewer positive emotions afterwards and are also more dissatisfied with their own body image than people who look at less attractive users.'[36] While Facebook and Twitter undoubtedly have negative effects on the user, Instagram was discovered to be the most mentally damaging social media network of all by #StatusofMind, a 2017 report published by the Royal Society for Public Health. They reported that the platform scored the lowest marks for health and wellbeing, with anxiety, depression and body dysmorphia emerging as some of the key negative side effects.

We tend to compare ourselves to people around us in our IRL lives every day but this comparison is very much heightened on social media, where imagery is so heavily curated and edited and *only* the best sides of someone tend to be shown. The majority of the most-followed people on Instagram are singers, models, actresses and sports players – which is problematic when you consider that, as a collective, they are very far from a true representation of society. Not only does how they look often have something to do with the reason they are so famous in the first place – due to how all-pervasive beauty standards are, for many of them it's important for their brand to look a certain way – they also work extremely hard to maintain their appearance using their ample means: think personal trainers, personal chefs, make-up artists and even surgery.

But it isn't just 'flawless' (by society's standard) pictures of celebrities and models that we're constantly subjected to, but also our friends and family . . . This is particularly troubling because it *feels* genuine; you're aware, when looking at a picture of a model or a celebrity that there's likely to be things like hair stylists, make-up artists, photographers and retouching involved, but when it's a photo of someone we know in real life, you think you're looking at a truly authentic photo. But even images posted by non-celebrities and non-models undergo a rigorous selection process – we all know how many shots it takes to get that perfect selfie! – followed by filtering and, more often than I bet you imagine, editing. Editing apps to change your body size and smooth your skin are so commonplace nowadays that I believe you might struggle to find many photos that are completely unretouched.

The result is that every single scroll provides ample opportunity to feel inadequate. I know this because I used to only follow people who conformed to the mainstream, traditional standard of beauty. Thin, tall women with long, luscious hair and curves in all the 'right' places. Why? Two reasons, the first one being that it wasn't until recently that the body positivity and body acceptance movements really came to light on social media; prior to their rise in popularity, not many people who fell outside of this standard showed off their bodies online. But it was also because I had been conditioned to believe that only one type of person (the thin, tall woman with long luscious hair and curves in all the 'right' places) was beautiful and, furthermore, that being beautiful like this was to be my eternal quest because beauty equalled happiness, success, desirability and worth.

My feed was chock full of women who I wanted to look like (but, crucially, never could). They were, I thought, serving as my 'inspiration' and 'motivation' – two words which are, it turns out, very much associated with pro-anorexia content – but in reality, they were leading me further and further away from self-acceptance and genuine happiness. The feelings of inadequacy each scroll brought up forced me into more dangerous territory – maybe if I could just lose a bit more, my stomach would be flat like that Victoria's Secret angel? Maybe if I buy that expensive in-clinic cellulite treatment package I will have smooth, lean thighs like that stunning Instagram model?

(I did this, by the way, and, spoiler alert, it didn't do a thing.) It fuelled my pre-existing insecurities until they were so heightened that I felt beyond uncomfortable in my body, like I wanted to crawl out of my own skin and just . . . be someone else. I felt, very deeply, that I simply wasn't enough.

When I first discovered plus-size models like Iskra Lawrence and Ashley Graham on Instagram, I was totally taken aback. I had never seen bodies that didn't fit the typical 'ideal' so unapologetically on display before – it was both refreshing and shocking. I feel guilty for saying I was shocked because they were just pictures of women's bodies – and ones that are still deemed 'acceptable', meaning that they do not face any discrimination or oppression for the way they look.

But that's what a lifetime of conditioning looks like, and I imagine you will have had the same reaction when you first started following people like me, for example. Again, even though my body is not marginalised (I am white and straight-sized), it's not the 'standard' body that is shown off so proudly. Usually those belong only to models and a very, very small percentage of the population. But just as conditioning is powerful, so is deconditioning.

I slowly began to curate my feed, unfollowing those who induced feelings of inadequacy and seeking out a more diverse range of people. I followed some who looked like me and others who didn't: people of all different shapes, sizes, races, genders and abilities. I was surprised at how quickly I became used to seeing this diverse range of bodies and, more importantly, how I was able to see the beauty in them. Rather than seeing them as imperfect, which is how society views anything outside of its definition of beauty, I was appreciating their bodies.

This, in turn, prompted me to look for the beauty in the bodies around me in real life and, crucially, my own. Which, after a lifetime of believing that my body was bad, that there was something wrong with it, felt incredibly liberating. And, while social media wasn't the only component in this process, it played a huge, and vital, part.

Because of this, when I talk to women in my Instagram DMs and answer the frequent question of 'How can I feel better about my body?', social media is often one of the first things I bring up. It's a crucial puzzle piece in the jigsaw we assemble that enables us to tackle negative body image created by diet culture. While other aspects of this process, like looking inwards to uncover and unpick longstanding self-limiting beliefs, can be very painful and energy draining (although absolutely imperative, don't get me wrong!), switching up your social media and filling your conscious and subconscious with more positive, inclusive messaging is a quick, easy and enjoyable way of increasing your self-esteem.

*But first up, we need to actually do it.*
*So let's curate the feed.*

For the time being, I'd love you to actively consider each account that pops up on your feed and evaluate how it makes you feel. Positive, inspired or uplifted? Are you able to relate and does it make you feel a little bit more comfortable in your own skin? Great. No action required.

If, on the other hand, the account induces any kind of negativity – whether that's sending you into a tailspin of negative thoughts, allowing self-doubt to creep in or prompting you to take inventory of your flaws – it's time to cull.

If one of these accounts happens to be someone you know and you're worried that unfollowing may cause resentment, the mute button is your friend – you can mute an account's post and/or stories, and they will never be any the wiser! And don't feel guilty about doing it – your priority has to be your mental health.

Once you've done this, you can then seek to fill your feed with a diverse range of people so you can increase your visual exposure to bodies that are typically underrepresented in traditional media. Look at the accounts you're left with: how many are Black? How many are people of colour? How many are disabled? How many are queer? How many exist in fat bodies? Big, confronting questions that might feel uncomfortable but that are really important. We have to take an active approach to cultivating diversity in our feed, while also respecting the boundaries of the new creators we follow.

Changing up our feed is of benefit for us as individuals. Over time, being exposed to a wide range of bodies reminds us how varied, different and beautiful the human race is, far beyond the skewed 5 per cent of 'perfect' bodies represented by traditional media, and that can be instrumental in helping you to appreciate your own. But there's also a huge social advantage in that exposure to the experiences of others encourages empathy, compassion and, ultimately, social change. Listen to what these accounts have to say about discrimination and their lived experiences (if they choose to tell them) and amplify their voices.

Another advantage of a diverse social media feed is access to a like-minded community that can lead to a mutually beneficial relationship that can help support you on your journeys to a better body image. This can be especially helpful if you lack such support in your real life. To help you on your way, here are some of my top suggestions of people to follow:

| | | |
|---|---|---|
| @ameniesseibi | @jess_megan_ | @sydneylbell |
| @antidietriotclub | @katiesturino | @tessholliday |
| @beauty_redefined | @kenziebrenna | @thebirdspapaya |
| @bodyimagewithbri | @khal_essie | @thebodzilla |
| @busybee_carys | @luuudaw | @thenutritiontea |
| @calliethorpe | @lvernon2000 | @tiffanyima |
| @curvynyome | @meg.boggs | @wheelchair_ |
| @dietitiananna | @miakang | rapunzel |
| @em_clarkson | @raindovemodel | @yourbodyisworthy |
| @emilylucyrajch | @sianlord_ | @yrfatfriend |
| @fullbodiedbekah | @sofiehagendk | @_nelly_london |
| @i_weigh | @sophjbutler | |
| @jaimmykoroma | @stephanieyeboah | |

Start with this digital detox straight away and your social media feed will soon become a beacon of positivity, rather than a space that endlessly encourages us to strive for unrealistic change.

I want to share a DM with you that, believe it or not, I received as I was writing this chapter. It's from a woman who messaged me a while back asking for help with feeling better about her own body. I encouraged her to review who she was following and supplied her with some suggestions. She came back to me with this feedback that I screenshotted immediately because I think it perfectly sums up what we're trying to achieve here:

> *'So much progress has been made since the last time we spoke. I've learnt so much from following you and the other people you have shared. It's so powerful that I've been able to better my body image through Instagram, the exact platform that contributed to destroying it. Thank you.'*

While taking stock of your online space is a fairly straightforward and simple way to improve your body image, being mindful of your *offline* space throws up many more challenges – we can't just mute or unfollow a family member, friend or colleague who we often have to spend time with.

We've all been subject to body shaming, right? Sometimes this comes from strangers but often, it's from people in our social or family circle. I have countless examples but there are a few that really stuck: being told at age 14 that I shouldn't be wearing short shorts anymore because of cellulite (at the very start of a day-long trip when I didn't have anything to change into); being steered towards tankinis rather than bikinis because 'they will suit your shape better' by a shop attendant and, most mortifying of all, overhearing a boy tell his friends I had a 'body that blocks out the sun' on my first-ever friends-only holiday at 17. I ran straight to my hotel room and locked myself in the bathroom, crying as I pinched my fat in the mirror. I stayed as covered up as the clothes in my suitcase would allow for the remainder of the trip.

Other highlights include being told I had legs 'like a footballer', which 'isn't nice for girls' and that I would be 'so pretty' if I could just get to a size 12 – you know, the classic 'you'd be so pretty if you lost weight' line.

Those kind of comments are crushing. They exist, of course, as a result of the perpetrator's own conditioning – we are all victims, at the end of the day – but they really hurt, especially if they're made by someone we love, and I'm so sorry if you've been on the receiving end of them. I understand the pain and just how destabilising it can be.

## So how can we handle them?

I don't believe that there's any one correct way to respond to hurtful body shaming comments or comments about our appearance – and a lot depends on context and what feels most comfortable to you. We're going to go into a few potential responses but I need to first make it clear that this is your body, your business – nobody else's. So when someone comments on it and it hurts you, you have every right to react in a way that feels right for you (I mean, maybe violence aside . . . !) and clearly set your boundaries.

Being British and predisposed to avoiding confrontation of any kind – it makes me incredibly flustered and I can't properly articulate what I need to say – the way that feels right to me is to give myself a bit of space, collect my thoughts, compose what I'd like to convey and send it in a message afterwards.

Here are a few other options:

- **Respond with a compliment:** I know, it sounds odd – bear with me. This is for the people who are intentionally trying to hurt your feelings. Choosing not to receive the comment and taking the higher ground by offering up a compliment in return is powerful: it's unexpected and jarring to the commenter and the dynamic instantly shifts; they are then left feeling guilty about their inappropriate remark.

- **Bat the comment straight back to them:** If you don't feel like being the better person (and god knows I very often don't), say 'so do you' and smile sweetly. Again, jarring and also, you know, a taste of their own medicine.

- **Call them out:** If you're up to it, stand strong and tell them what they said was inappropriate, that *your* body is none of *their* business and demand that they never pass comment on your or anybody else's body/weight/eating every again. You have every right to do this.

- **Ignore it:** I find this too difficult, personally, but not giving a reaction at all is a powerful way to stop a bodyshamer – especially one that has the sole intention of provoking a reaction – in their tracks.

- **Remove yourself:** If you've cycled through these possible options and the body shaming continues, it might be worth considering removing yourself from the line of fire and cutting ties with that particular person. This isn't always a possibility but if it is, it's worth contemplating: truly looking after and out for yourself includes taking yourself away from potentially damaging situations.

It's not just negative comments that are difficult to respond to; knowing how to handle seemingly positive comments or compliments about weight loss can also be tricky. Quick experiment: raise your hand if you've ever said: 'Wow, you've lost weight – you look amazing!' Yeah, same. I've done it so many times in the past.

It's usually well intentioned because we're conditioned to believe that weight loss = good, weight gain = bad and thinness is to be celebrated above all else. But this is a myth that actively causes harm – and congratulating people for losing weight with a compliment for how they now look perpetuates that harm. These kind of comments can impact our self-esteem as it reinforces the idea that we're better when we're thinner and that there was something wrong with our body previously.

When someone offers us something they believe is a compliment, it's difficult to say anything but 'thank you', simply because it's hammered into us to be thankful for compliments to the point that it's practically a reflex reaction.

And yes, sometimes weight loss is the goal, whether for health reasons or other personal reasons, and you might welcome the compliment. I totally understand that – society has made us believe that we need to be thin so when someone praises you for it, it feels good – but I think it's really important to understand that the compliment still serves to perpetuate fatphobia and diet culture by implying that thinner is better.

Often, weight loss is not intentional: it can be as a result of stress, poor mental health, medication or bereavement, alongside a whole host of other reasons. In these cases, the compliment is even more icky. Commenting on other people's bodies at all is off, let's face it, even if it is well intentioned.

Not responding when someone remarks on your weight loss positively with 'thank you' is difficult but so important. Here are some other possible retorts:

- 'I know you mean well, but when you praise my weight loss, it makes me feel like who I was before wasn't good enough.'

- 'I actually feel a bit uncomfortable with that because weight loss hasn't been a goal of mine.'

- 'I'm actually going through a really stressful time right now; how my body looks is the last thing on my mind.'

- 'I have lost weight, yes, but that hasn't impacted me in any other way apart from appearance!'

- 'Yes, I have, but unfortunately, that hasn't been positive for me.'

You could also just shrug and change the subject – whatever you're most comfortable with. This isn't prescriptive; I just want to offer you some options.

What people think
of you is none of
your business.

Above all, I need you to know, with full certainty, that their comments mean everything about them and nothing about you; it's a projection of their own issues and insecurities. Because why should how our bodies look affect anyone else? It shouldn't, because it doesn't – it doesn't affect their wellbeing, their health or their life.

An incredible piece of advice I was given by my friend Emily Clarkson, while I was reeling from the unkind words of a troll on Instagram, is that what people think of you is none of your business. It took me a while to fully understand this and, don't get me wrong, it's something that I still sometimes have trouble fully believing when I feel triggered by words, but it's so true: your own thoughts and your own actions are the only thing you can control. And, as Marcus Aurelius said: 'The happiness of your life depends on the quality of your thoughts.' Obsessing over what someone else thinks about you takes away control of your own thoughts.

The journey to self-acceptance is often long and difficult, especially if you are starting from a place of damage or difficulty, thanks to eating disorders or simply the distorted view of bodies sold to us by diet culture. We may not be able to control what others say to us but we have the power to choose what we let into our space via social media and we can control our responses to any comments we do receive. So curate your space the best that you can and try to focus on the fact that so much of what people say to us is about *them*, not us. I truly believe that this is the best way to build up armour that shields us from negativity and allows us to continue on our path to making peace with ourselves and finding true happiness.

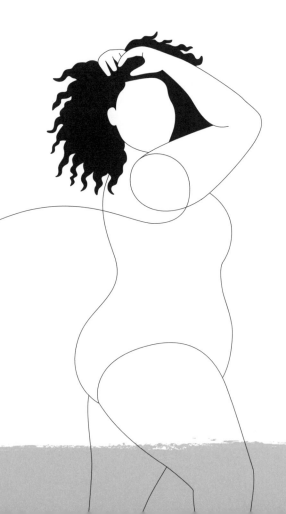

# CHAPTER 13

# The windy road forward: where to go from here

So, here
we are!
How are you
feeling?

Hopefully excited at the possibility of living a life without hating your body – but maybe a bit overwhelmed. I get it, it's a lot.

And you don't have to go at it all at once. Admittedly, I'm very all-or-nothing in my mentality, so if I were reading this book, I'd probably try to implement every single bit of advice straight away . . . It's all I'd do and think about for a few weeks and then I'd end up burning out. Don't be like me – take it one step at a time and give yourself space to digest and understand. If necessary, read the entire book again, or just certain chapters. There's a lot to process and internalise – and a lot of it goes against everything we thought we knew. Afford yourself compassion.

I'm also guilty of looking for a quick fix, so I might hyper-fixate on one certain area. For example, I would probably come across the intuitive eating chapter, think I've had a 'light-bulb' moment (you know – the 'this is going to be it! This is going to sort EVERYTHING!' moment) and throw myself into intuitive eating. But while intuitive eating will likely eventually help you heal your relationship with food, you still need to work on fixing your relationship with your body image, too, which requires understanding and dismantling diet culture on a personal level, having knowledge about fatphobia and beauty standards and challenging existing self-beliefs about your weight and value in this world.

I must say, though I have been quite prone to it in the past, I'm not a huge fan of the 'light-bulb moment'/turning point concept. I'd heard many eating disorder recoverers say that they experienced a pivotal moment that marked the imminent end point of their recovery, but this was detrimental to me because

I was always looking for *mine*. I was constantly waiting for my 'aha' moment but it never came, so I thought I wasn't progressing.

But the truth, I believe, is that progress is much more complex and lengthy than one single defining moment. I describe my recovery – both from an eating disorder and from severely negative body image – as imperceptible bits of growth that gradually stacked up on top of each other to form real, perceptible progress. It's not really as exciting a story or sexy an answer as 'I woke up one day and realised I couldn't do this anymore and that was pretty much it!', is it?!

It's a cliché but I can't stress it enough and I *need* you to know: this road is not linear – you'll have ups, downs, steps forward and steps backward. You'll have days where you're doing so well that you think you've done it, you've made peace with your body, and then you'll have days where you feel so consumed by negative thoughts that you think you might be back at square one.

Try to stay away from this black-and-white thinking – rather than believe that your journey is complete on the good days and that your journey hasn't even began on the bad days, try to move to a grey area. Acknowledge that you have made progress and congratulate yourself on that progress, but appreciate that you still have a way to go – and that's absolutely fine.

Setbacks are difficult. I distinctly remember a time when I feeling very confident and happy in my own skin – it was beyond joyful, I felt deliriously happy. I was visiting my parents in Cyprus and I was wearing bikinis without a second thought; my body was having absolutely no negative impact

on my mind whatsoever – an incredible feeling after spending
a lifetime at war with it. While I was out there, I went to see a
dermatologist for a problem I was having with my skin. When
the dermatologist asked me if I was taking any tablets, I told
him I was taking medication for my acid reflux (sexy and I
know it but beside the point). He proceeded to tell me – you
can guess what's coming, can't you?! – that he knew what the
cure was. Weight loss! 'You need to lose some weight. Lose five
to ten kilos by going on a low calorie diet,' he said. 'You need
to balance your weight and your acid reflux will disappear.'

I was stunned; I left in silence, dazed by what I had just been
told. It wasn't until afterwards that I wished, so badly, that I
had stood my ground and told him how damaging advising
his patients (who were visiting for a skin condition!) to lose
weight could be – especially because an eating disorder is the
most likely culprit of my acid reflux in the first place – but I
felt too dumbstruck to formulate anything coherent.

And just like that, my confidence was crushed. I felt humiliated
and suddenly self-conscious of my body, left wondering what
other people were thinking about me. I was frustrated at myself
for letting a random man who had no impact on my life derail
me with a few sentences but I couldn't deny it: he had. I felt like
I was back at square one, all progress scrapped.

But as the days passed, I started to feel stronger. I realised a few
things: that man was wrapped up in the diet culture belief that
everyone needs to be a certain (low) weight to be healthy; he was
simply reverting to weight loss as a cure for something he didn't
fully understand (I know that weight loss can sometimes aid acid

reflux, but it's not weight-related for me) because it's what he learnt in medical school and, most importantly, it didn't matter what that man thought of me and my body. What matters is what *I* think of me and my body, and I can't afford to pass that power to anyone else. Plus, nobody else deserves that power. I actually came out of this setback stronger – and armed with new tools to help me cope effectively with something similar should it arise again.

What I'm trying to get at is this: those setbacks – whether it's someone commenting on your body, trying on a pair of jeans that don't fit or seeing pictures of yourself that you don't like – that make you feel despondent and discouraged? It does not mean you've failed in your journey and it doesn't mean you haven't made progress.

Actually, I believe those little lapses are critical to our progress: they are where we gather more tools with which to arm ourselves, so we come back stronger. The next time we fall down, so to speak, we're then able to pick ourselves up much quicker.

Living in this appearance-obsessed world, it's unrealistic to think that you will never have bad body image days. I have pretty much done as much work as anyone can to improve my body image and, while most days I don't even give my appearance a second thought, there are still days where I don't feel so great in my own skin. I reach for baggier clothing and refrain from having any photos taken of me.

The difference now is that I have the right weapons in my arsenal to get myself back to a good place as soon as possible.

Here are some examples:

- **I afford myself compassion**. It's normal to have bad body image days and I don't try to snap myself out of it.

- Instead, **I lean into the emotions with curiosity**, with the aim of exploring why it is that I'm not feeling so great in my body. For example, if I have rejection in an area of my life – let's say a work rejection – I start feeling not so good in my body. Because that's always been my default mode of punishment when I'm feeling rejected. This curiosity helps you identify and understand your triggers, meaning you can both set boundaries to avoid such triggers AND work through the triggers to get to a point of neutrality. Ultimately, it makes you realise that it's not about your body.

- **I make time for self-care**. Often, the negative feelings around my body are because I'm lacking a bit of self-TLC, so I allow myself to do something that I love doing, like watching a good few episodes of a *Real Housewives* show (my favourite) or do a full skincare routine and paint my nails. Self-care is different for everyone, so opt for things that feel good for you and remind yourself to take care of YOU.

- **I make sure to move my body.** I find this to be a really powerful way to shift my mindset from how my body looks to how it feels – and what it's capable of. You can choose any movement you like – remember, it doesn't have to be gruelling and it's not about changing your body!

- **I take a scroll**. I follow so many incredible, inspirational people that consistently share nuggets of wisdom, so when I'm feeling not-so-good, I scroll through my Insta feed and start to feel my mood lift.

- **I try to always challenge negative self-talk**. I think that while it's important to let the negative emotions rise up and be explored, it's equally as important to challenge them and remind yourself that you don't deserve cruel words.

What can be very helpful on these more difficult days is to get a piece of paper and make two columns: one to write down your reasons to want to improve your body image and the other to note your progress so far – even the tiniest bits, everything. I have a notebook almost entirely dedicated to this because it was so useful in reminding me why I needed to be on this journey and all of my achievements along the way (it's easy to forget when you're in a darker space). Every time, this exercise would help to lift my spirits and renew my determination.

I want you to remember, above all, that while you might be having a bad body image day, that does not mean that you have a bad body, as my friend Nelly London once said. Because despite the term 'body image', the problem doesn't actually lie with the body – it's all about the mind. I find this to be perfectly illustrated by a quote, the author of which, unfortunately, I can't seem to be able to identify, but here it is: 'You know when you look back at an old photo of you and think, "Wow, why did I hate my body then?" – THAT'S your proof that it has never been about your body.'

You know when you look back at an old photo of you and think, 'Wow, why did I hate my body then?'

– THAT'S your proof that it has never been about your body.

This is one of the most powerful quotes I've ever read – and, funnily enough, reading it was as close to a light-bulb moment as I've ever had . . . That photo from ten years ago when I felt like I wanted to crawl out of my own skin because I felt so disgusting? I looked great. Why was I *so* uncomfortable? It wasn't anything to do with my body, it was everything to do with my *perception* of my body. A very important distinction.

In ten years' time, I don't want to be looking back at photos of myself now and thinking the same thing. Ideally, I won't be thinking about how I look at *all* – but we live in a world that makes that near impossible, so I at least want to be thinking: 'I looked great then and I look great now, and I'm so happy I've spent the last ten years not allowing how I look to hold me back from living life.'

I want to touch on why I mentioned that in an ideal world, I wouldn't be thinking about how I looked, and I want to use quotes from Dr Lindsay Kite and Dr Lexie Kite, co-authors of *More Than a Body*, from one of their posts on Instagram @beauty_redefined: 'Most people think body confidence is rooted in accepting how you look. That's why body positivity influencers are so popular – they show and tell you how confident they are in their looks so you can feel good, too. This is a first step toward body confidence for lots of people, but it is not the only step.'

'Your body is not an object to be looked at, so healing your body image – your perception and feelings about your body – is not about changing how you *view* your body; it's about changing how you *value* your body. If your body confidence comes from liking how you look, it will rise and fall with every nice or negative comment, every acceptance or rejection, every good or bad photo, and every physical and mental fluctuation. It can also fall when your #bopo inspos lose weight or get cosmetic surgery or express dissatisfaction with their bodies that look just like yours. If she doesn't actually feel as good as she seemed to, how could you be expected to?'

This was illustrated recently by Adele's weight loss. Adele was once viewed as a fat heroine, representing plus-size women across the world who suddenly felt less alone by seeing a bigger girl reach so much fame and adoration. But then she lost weight and it was really triggering for many of those women. Adele made them feel more accepted by showing that if she could be proud of her body, they could be proud of theirs, too. Her weight loss felt like that permission to be comfortable in their own skin was snatched away, replaced by a desire to lose weight to receive praise and admiration. (Adele caused a global frenzy in 2020 when her weight loss was first revealed, with thousands of news outlet praising her 'amazing transformation' and speculating about how she managed to lose the weight. The first thing that appears when you start typing 'Adele' into Google is still 'Adele weight loss' and if you google 'Adele weight', there are over 75 million results.)

But how can those women – and people who experience similar triggers – move past this? Lindsay and Lexie explain that true body confidence is learning to value your body as an instrument for your use – not an ornament to be admired. Again, this isn't an easy thing to accomplish overnight, especially in the diet culture and patriarchy-dominated society in which we exist, and it's not a one-time accomplishment that is done for life, but their work in body image resilience illustrates that it is achievable and life-changing. They write, 'You may feel ashamed about how you look at times and sometimes lament the ways in which your body might fall shorts in terms of abilities, health and/or expectations. And that's OK – it's going to happen, be kind to yourself when it does. But rather than pushing that shame deep down and attempting to rebuild confidence by "improving" your body, these moments of shame can serve as your action moments. Let them be your reminder of how urgent it is to see more in yourself and your body – more than an object to be fixed and judged – and act accordingly. You can come back to your body as your home instead of self-objectifying and dividing against yourself.'

Some of the practical tips the Kites discuss in *More Than a Body* in order to achieve this include:

- Reflect on the unfair pressure and distorted messages about beauty and worth that have contributed to your pain.

- Express compassion to yourself as you consciously root out those sources of objectification in your life and ask others to join you in healing and growing as more than a body.

- Extend that kindness to those you'd normally judge, police or compare yourself to.

- Prioritise how you live over how you look. Prioritise how you experience the world over how the world experiences you.

- Ask yourself – what do I really want to do, feel, achieve and experience in and through this body of mine? Whatever it is you want to do and be, try it. Regardless of how you look or what think you need to qualify. Just try.

Again, it's a lot to take in. Especially for a mind, like mine, that's impatient . . . I remember, during one of my many breakdowns to my husband Dave, saying to him: 'Nothing's working, I can't do this! All this work and I don't even feel any better.' As he tried to console me – this man deserves a medal – he came up with an analogy that stuck with me and actually helped guide me from there on out.

He compared the process of making peace with your body to a jigsaw puzzle. The individual parts don't mean much at all, and they're confusing to look at, but when they come together, they form something. The image becomes clearer and clearer the more pieces of the puzzle that you add, until eventually you can see the whole picture. It was working, I had made progress, I just needed a few more pieces of the puzzle. So simple, and so powerful, right?

Speaking of Dave, I have to discuss the importance of opening up to someone. It is so hard to suffer in silence. And you shouldn't have to – you deserve support. I was incredibly secretive about my disordered eating and eating disorders (until I decided to share it with the world, apparently?!) and it did me no good. It was, in fact, harmful: it allowed my issues to progress and become further ingrained without intervention. But I was too consumed with shame. When I eventually told my mum and dad what was going on, it was the start of me getting help – they were so understanding and so desperate to help me get better that I was lucky enough to start treatment almost straight away.

Then, later down the line when I was still suffering, I opened up to Dave. I was nervous and scared, but it was getting to a point where I had no choice but to tell him because it was impacting my life so heavily. I had no idea how he would react but I needn't have worried: he was kind, compassionate and understanding – remarkably, given he's never really had any kind of body image or eating issues himself. His unwavering support – I must have had the same breakdown to him at least 100 times and I don't think this is an exaggeration – and constant compassion helped to eventually pull me through one of the darkest times of my life. I hope I don't sound like I'm bragging, I know that I was very lucky to have such an understanding partner and caring parents, but I want to stress just how important it is to receive support. Things like this – learning to be comfortable in your own skin after a lifetime of hating it – are much easier to cope with when you have someone you can offload to and confide in. Someone who hears how you feel and is there for you to lean on when it all feels too overwhelming.

I'd recommend opening up to someone you feel might understand. It's true that some people just won't get it, and that's not necessarily their fault. Not everyone is able to be as emotionally intelligent and understanding with these issues as you need. So think about who might be the best person, who feels like a 'safe person'. Maybe a friend that you trust implicitly, or your mum, or your sister. These are just examples – you know who is right for you.

If your body dissatisfaction leads to you engaging in self-destructive behaviours, telling someone can also hold you accountable. An example of this was when I was trying to escape the clutches of bulimia. Dave suggested I contact him every time I wanted to purge. It was a hugely generous offer. I agreed, and that became integral to eventually overcoming the bulimia.

I've encouraged people to open up to someone they trust many, many times, and, often, they come back and tell me that the person they confided in revealed they are actually going through something similar. More of us suffer in silence than you think. Even the friend who you think is incredibly beautiful, or the one who is greatly admired by men, or even the model in the magazine – so many of these women still face body confidence issues, despite meeting society's standard of beauty: this does not negate such internal struggles. You're less alone than you may imagine.

You're less alone than
you may imagine.

I also need you to remember that it's vital that you extend compassion and kindness to yourself. I cannot stress enough how imperative it is to be kind to yourself. Negative self-talk will only breed negative emotions and negative actions; offering yourself compassion will make you feel safe and cared for and mentally more resilient. Not sure how to start? Try to talk to yourself like you would to a young child or someone you love when you want to soothe them. Practise catching critical thoughts and try to reframe them into more kind and loving comments. Look back at your 'progress' list and feel proud of everything you've accomplished so far. Give yourself credit.

And, above all, remember that life is too short to wait to live it until you fit into those jeans, or lose a certain amount of weight, or get rid of your cellulite. It's too short to live as a 'before' picture. You are not a 'before' picture and you're not an 'after' picture, either – and neither are any of those people from the transformation shots we see online. We are living, breathing, multi-faceted, talented human beings whose true beauty cannot be captured in a picture. A picture cannot convey someone's warmth and compassion, how they make people laugh, how they're loyal friends or the mark they've made on the world.

Our bodies are merely the vessels that hold all the good stuff. They were created for us to live out our purpose, so let's live it. And, as the famous quote goes,

*The best time to start was yesterday. The next best time is now.*

# FURTHER READING

Lindsay Kite PhD & Lexie Kite PhD, *More Than A Body* (2020)

Sabrina Strings, *Fearing The Black Body: The Racial Origins of Fat Phobia* (2020)

Christy Harrison, *Anti-Diet* (2019)

Stephanie Yeboah, *Fattily Ever After: A Black Fat Girl's Guide To Living Life Unapologetically* (2020)

Aubrey Gordon, *What We Don't Talk About When We Talk About Fat* (2020)

Dr Joshua Wolrich, *Food Isn't Medicine* (2021)

Tally Rye, *Train Happy: An Intuitive Exercise Plan For Every Body* (2020)

Laura Thomas, *Just Eat it* (2019)

Elyse Resch & Evelyn Tribole, *Intuitive Eating: A Revolutionary Program that Works* (2012)

Lindo Bacon, *Health At Every Size: The Surprising Truth About Your Weight* (2010)

Lindo Bacon PhD & Lucy Aphramore PhD, *Body Respect* (2014)

Molly Forbes, *Body Happy Kids* (2021)

Brené Brown, *The Gifts of Imperfection* (2020)

Naomi Wolf, *The Beauty Myth* (1990)

Katie Sturino, *Body Talk* (2021)

Rose Molinary, *Beautiful You* (2010)

Jessica Sanders, *Love Your Body* (2019)

Poorna Bell, *Stronger* (2021)

Kelsey Miller, *Big Girl: How I Gave Up Dieting and Got a Life* (2016)

Jes Baker, *Landwhale* (2018)

# NOTES ON THE TEXT

**1** Poll commissioned by Love Berries UK: www.mirror.co.uk/news/uk-news/brits-try-126-fad-diets-21234747

**2** I have capitalised Black whenever I reference race, in recognition of the shared history and identity amongst everyone who identifies as Black across the world.

**3** F. R. E. Smink, Daphne van Hoeken and Hans W. Hoek, 'Epidemiology of Eating Disorders: Incidence, Prevalence and Mortality Rates', *Current Psychiatry Reports* (Aug 2012), 14(4), 406–14.

**4** Traci Mann, A. J. Tomiyama, Erika Westling, Ann-Marie Lew, Barbara Samuels and Jason Chatman, 'Medicare's search for effective obesity treatments: diets are not the answer', *American Psychologist* (Apr 2007), 62(3), 220–33.

**5** K. H. Pietiläinen, S. E. Saarni, J. Kaprio and A. Rissanen, 'Does dieting make you fat? A twin study', *International Journal of Obesity* (Mar 2012), 36(3), 456–64.

**6** Leah M. Kalm and Richard D. Semba, 'They starved so that others be better fed: remembering Ancel Keys and the Minnesota experiment', *Journal of Nutrition* (Jun 2005), 135(6), 1347–52.

**7** Evelyn Tribole and Elyse Resch, *Intuitive Eating: An Anti-Diet Revolutionary Approach* (4th edition, St. Martin's Essentials, 2020).

**8** Figures from www.ceros.com/inspire/originals/fashion-magazine-covers-diversity-media/

**9** Patricia Van den Berg, Dianne Neumark-Sztainer, Peter J. Hannan and Jess Haines, 'Is dieting advice from magazines helpful or harmful? Five-year associations with weight-control behaviors and psychological outcomes in adolescents', *Pediatrics* (Jan 2007), 119(1), e30–7.

**10** Grace Holland and Marika Tiggemann, 'A systematic review of the impact of the use of social networking sites on body image and disordered eating outcomes', *Body Image* (Jun 2016), 17, 100–110.

**11** Mario Palmer, '5 Facts About Body Image', *Amplify* (2013), quoted on https://www.dosomething.org/us/facts/11-facts-about-body-image.

**12** M. P. McCabe, L. A. Ricciardelli and J. Finemore, 'The role of puberty, media and popularity with peers on strategies to increase weight, decrease weight and increase muscle tone among adolescent boys and girls', *Journal of Psychosomatic Research* (Mar 2002), 52(3), 145–154.

**13** Sharon Hayes and Stacey Tantleff-Dunn, 'Am I too fat to be a princess? Examining the effects of popular children's media on young girls' body image', *British Journal of Developmental Psychology* (Jun 2010), 28(2), 413–426.

**14** Research carried out by Revealing Reality, commissioned by the 5Rights Foundation, which campaigns for tighter online controls for children.

**15** Norman Sartorius, 'The Meanings of Health and its Promotion', *Croatian Medical Journal* (Aug 2006), 47(4), 662–64.

**16** Sabina Strings, *Fearing The Black Body: The Racial Origins of Fat Phobia*, (NYU Press, 2019).

**17** Linda Bacon, *Health at Every Size: The Surprising Truth About Your Weight* (2nd edition, BenBella Books, 2010).

**18** *Journal of the American Medical Association* (2013).

**19** https://rugbyroar.com/what-is-the-average-size-of-a-rugby-player/

**20** Katherine M. Flegal, Brian K. Kit, Heather Orpana and Barry Graubard, 'Association of all-cause mortality with overweight and obesity using standard body mass index categories: a systematic review and meta-analysis', *Journal of the American Medical Association* (Jan 2013), 309(1), 71–82.

**21** 2018 data from the British Liver Trust.

**22** Timothy A. Judge and Daniel M. Cable, 'When it comes to pay, do the thin win? The effect of weight on pay for men and women', *Journal of Applied Psychology* (Jan 2011), 96(1), 95–112.

**23** A. R. Sutin, Y. Stephan and A. Terracciano, 'Weight discrimination and risk of mortality', *Psychological Science* (Nov 2015), 26(11), 1803–11.

**24** Jon Arcelus, Alex J. Mitchell, Jackie Wales, Søren Nielsen, 'Mortality rates in patients with anorexia nervosa and other eating disorders. A meta-analysis of 36 studies', *Archives of General Psychiatry* (Jul 2011), 68(7), 724–31.

**25** Study published in *The British Medical Journal*. Data was collected from the General Practice Research Database.

**26** Survey from the International Society of Aesthetic Plastic Surgery on the continuing rise in aesthetic surgery worldwide. Accessed at: https://www.isaps.org/wp-content/uploads/2020/12/ISAPS-Global-Survey-2019-Press-Release-English.pdf.

**27** The Aesthetic Society, 'Aesthetic Plastic Surgery National Databank Statistics 2020'. Accessed at https://cdn.theaestheticsociety.org/media/statistics/aestheticplasticsurgerynationaldatabank-2020stats.pdf

**28** Abby Ellin, 'Brazilian Butt Lifts Surge, Despite Risks', *The New York Times* (19 Aug 2021).

**29** BAAPS statement on Brazilian Buttock Lifts. Accessed at https://baaps.org.uk/media/press_releases/1621/baaps_statement_on_brazilian_buttock_lifts

**30** Luis Rios, Jr, MD and Varun Gupta, MD, MPH, 'Improvement in Brazilian Butt Lift (BBL) Safety With the Current Recommendations from ASERF, ASAPS, and ISAPS', *The Aesthetic Surgery Journal* (April 2020), 1-7

**31** You can find her website at www.intuitivepsychologyacademy.com

**32** Lauren F Friedman, 'A psychologist reveals the biggest predictor of happiness — and it's not money', *Insider*, Sep 6, 2015. Accessed at https://www.businessinsider.com/how-to-know-you-are-happy-psychology-2015-9

**33** Stephen R. Swallow and Nicholas A. Kuiper, 'Social comparison in dysphoria and nondysphoria: Differences in target similarity and specificity', *Cognitive Therapy and Research* (1993), 17(2), 103–22.

**34** www.statista.com/statistics/507378/average-daily-media-use-in-the-united-kingdom-uk/

**35** Studies by The Florida House Experience, a mental health and addiction treatment facility. Accessed at: https://fherehab.com/news/bodypositive/

**36** Nina Haferkamp and Nicole C. Krämer, 'Social comparison 2.0: examining the effects of online profiles on social-networking sites', *Cyberpsychology, Behavior, and Social Networking* (May 2011), 14(5), 309–14.

# INDEX

# ACKNOWLEDGEMENTS

Well, wow – turns out writing a book is just as hard as people say it is! And entirely impossible (at least, for me) without an incredible team of people, so here goes . . .

First of all – because they'll kill me if I don't – I must thank my wonderful mum and dad, Norma and David Light, without whom none of this would be possible, for being the best and most supportive parents . . . even if my mum is still not entirely sure what I do 😌

In terms of the day-to-day making of this book, I honestly don't think I could have done it without my husband Dave. From endless encouragement and heaps of consolation as I hit multiple breaking points and flounced away from my laptop shouting 'I can't do this', to constant cups of tea and taking over my share of dog walks. You were (and still are) my rock.

Oh, and speaking of dogs, a big thank you to my gorgeous little hound Betty for providing me with instant calm and limitless cuddles during the aforementioned breakdowns.

At this point, my (four) sisters will be reading this and on the verge of sending a passive aggressive text saying 'erm, where is our mention????' so I'd better get to it. Jen, Katherine, Ellie and Sophie, thanks for all your help in sense-checking for this book, your discerning eyes and for being absolute legends in general. You all bring total chaos to my life, but I wouldn't have it any other way.

Is this turning into an Oscars speech? I knew it would.

I'd also like to thank my primary school netball teacher for . . . Just kidding, back to it.

I need to thank the entire team at Harper Collins HQ, with particular and huge thanks to my commissioning editor Zoë Berville – I'm forever grateful to you: not just for your hard work and patience, but also for taking a chance on me. You believed in this book way before I could ever let myself, and I still can't believe we're here – we did it!

Speaking of getting it done, an enormous thank you to my brilliant manager Will Prior at my agency 84 World – you were instrumental in making this book happen and I am so, so appreciative for your constant, unwavering support and belief in me . . . even when I'm driving you nuts. Which is often.

I must also thank Liz Marvin, who whipped my manuscript into tip top shape and fielded my rather extensive indecisiveness and uncertainty (like I said, writing a book is hard!) with grace and patience.

I want to shout out the people working behind the scenes to make this book a success: Louise Evans for bringing my vision to life with your stunning designs and illustrations; Abi and Millie for your keen editorial eyes and thoughtful input; Dawn Burnett and Lily Capewell for working hard to get the word out about it with your PR and marketing genius; Halema Begum in the Production team for ensuring that it looks absolutely stunning; and Georgina Green, Harriet Williams, Ange Thomson, Sara Eusebi and Darren Shoffren for making sure people actually buy it . . . !

Another thank you goes to my brilliant friend Hannah Walters-Wood, who has always been on the other end of the phone for expert help and sense-checking with writing and design, and my assistant Amy Sadler for holding the fort while I got.this.done.

*music starts to play me off stage . . .*

And last, but far from least – you guys. I would never be here without your support and I just hope you know how much I appreciate it. For all its pitfalls, Instagram has given me this incredible community that has not only helped me recover from my eating disorder and reframe how I see my body, but uplifted me and given me purpose . . . I no longer see the years of my life I spent in the thick of eating disorders as wasted, because it has brought me to this, and to you. Thank you.

*dragged off stage*